Radiation Oncology

Edited by Badruddeen, Usama Ahmad, Mohd Aftab Siddiqui and Juber Akhtar

Published in London, United Kingdom

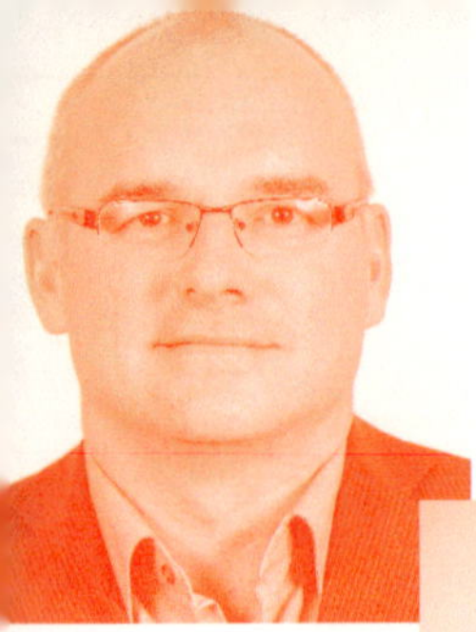
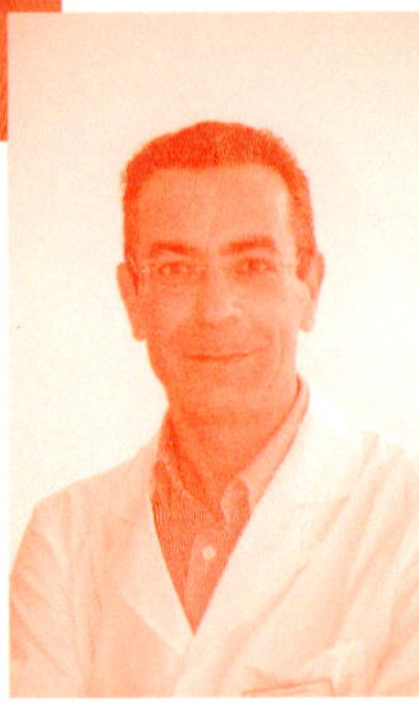
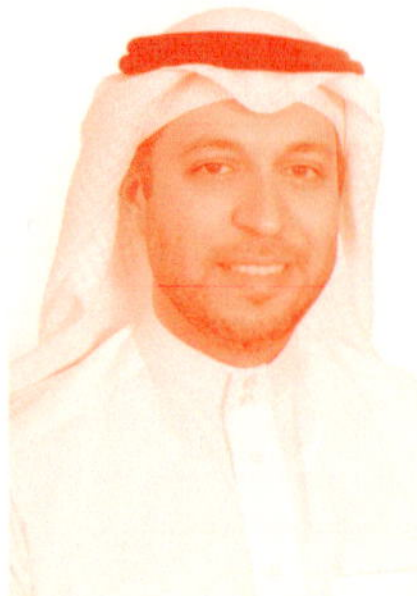
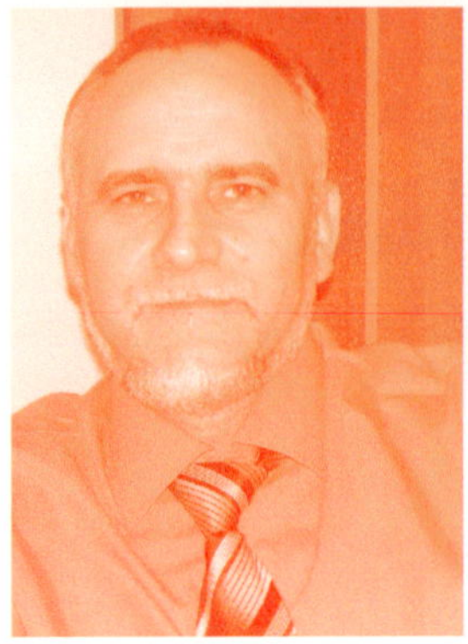
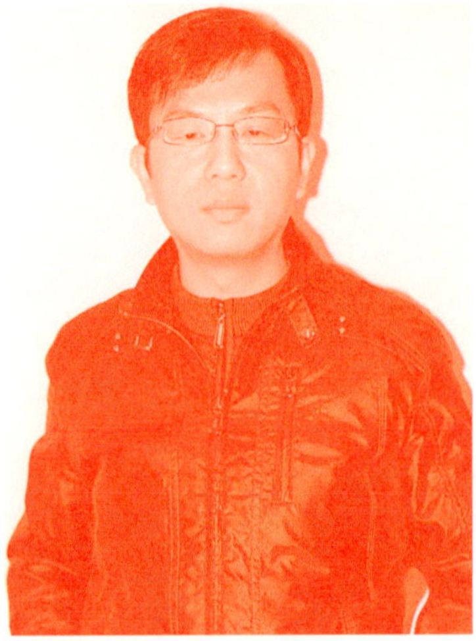
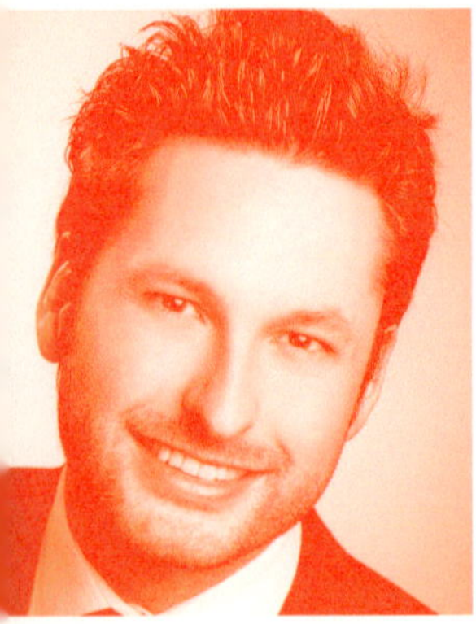
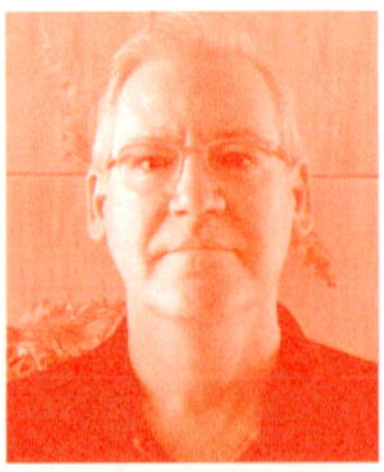

IntechOpen

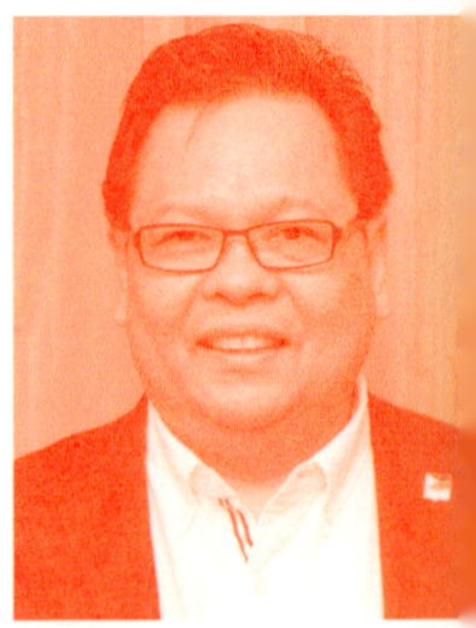
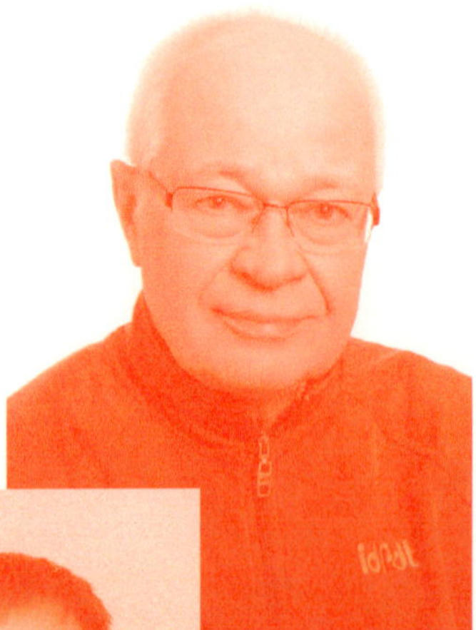
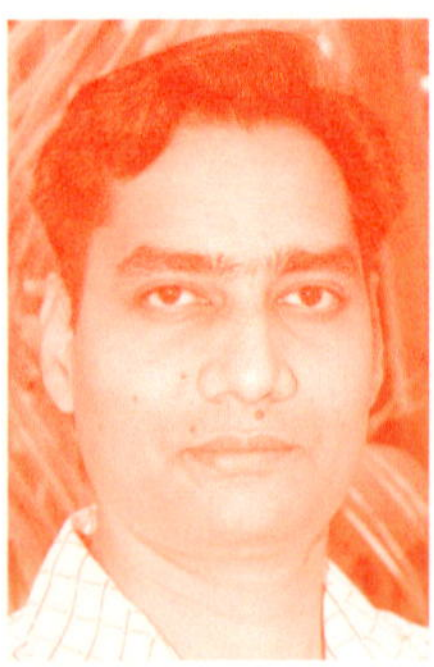
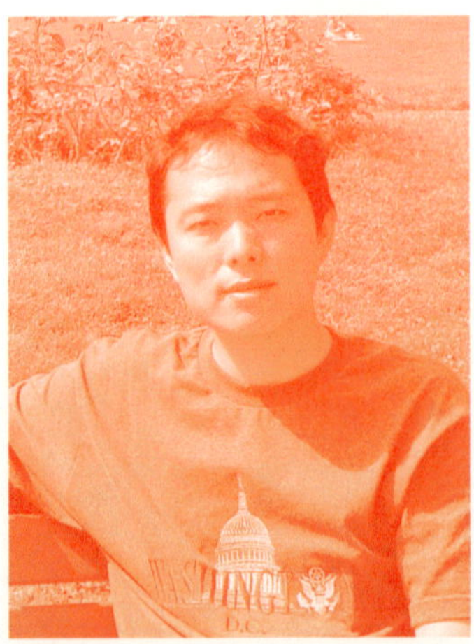
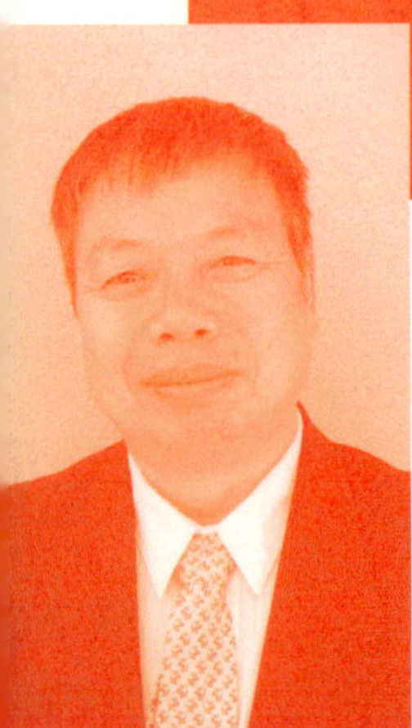
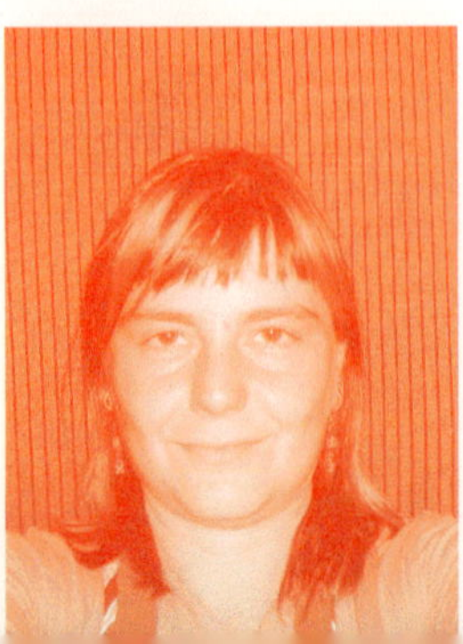

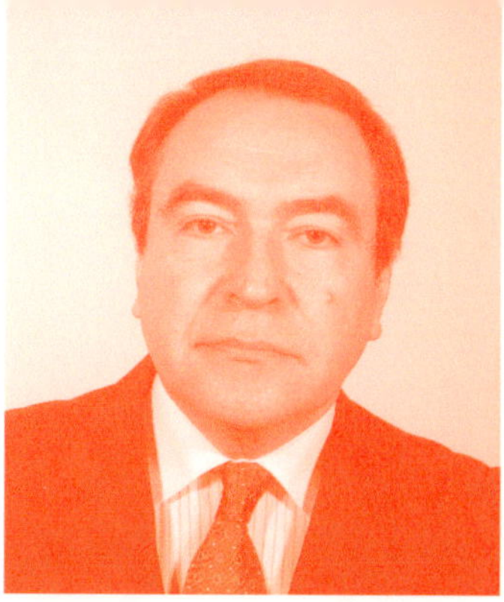

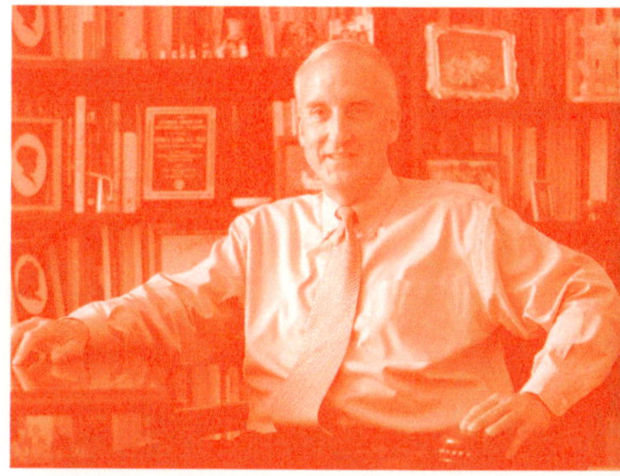

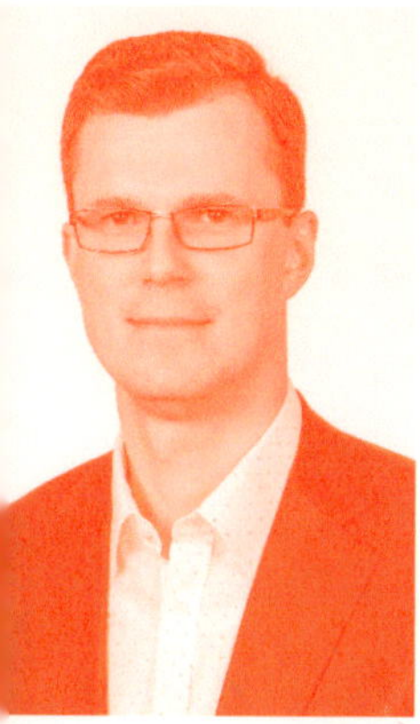

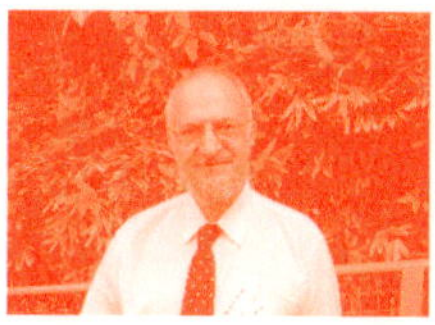

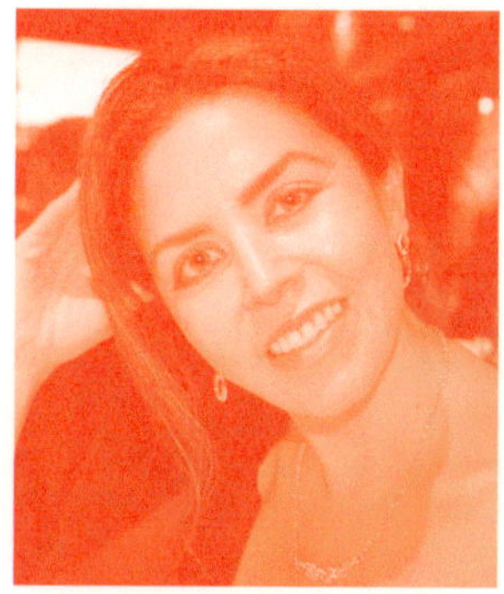

Supporting open minds since 2005

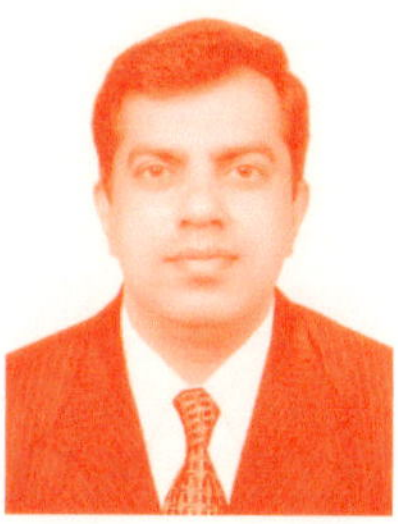

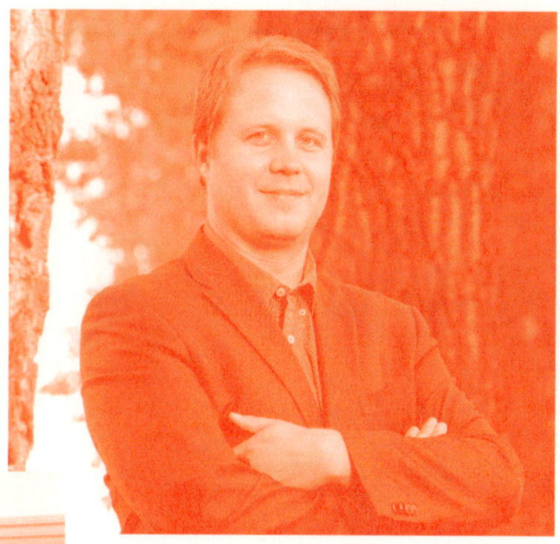

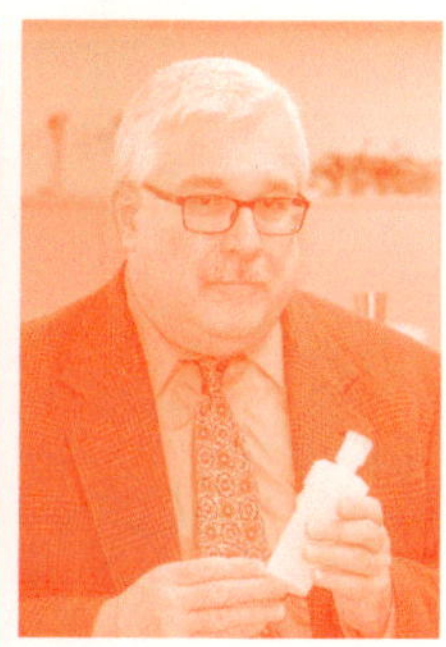

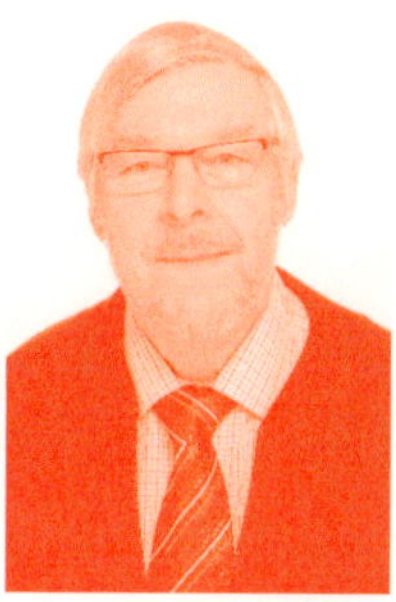

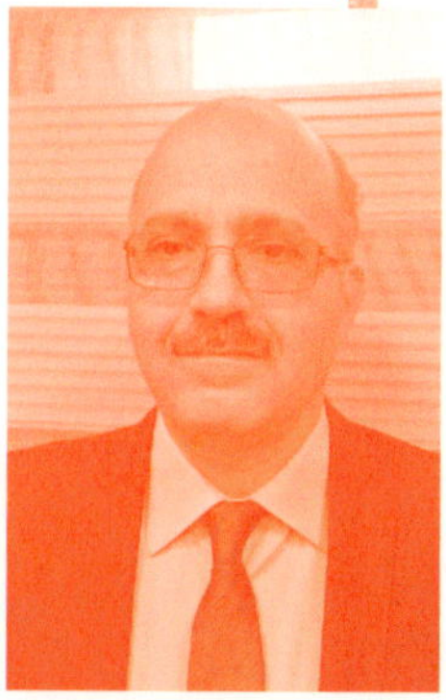

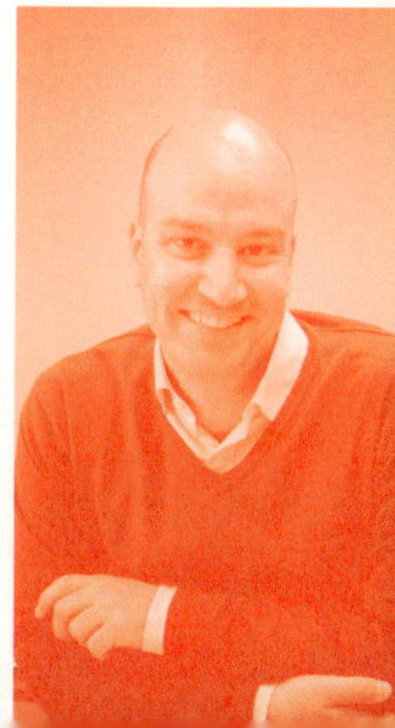

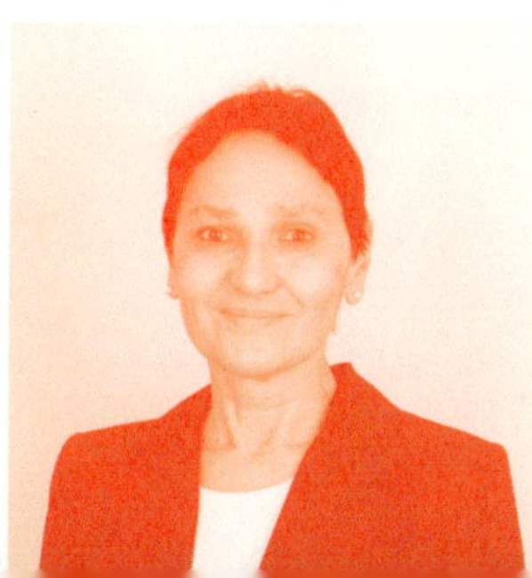

Radiation Oncology
http://dx.doi.org/10.5772/intechopen.94818
Edited by Badruddeen, Usama Ahmad, Mohd Aftab Siddiqui and Juber Akhtar

Contributors
Katia Manolova Sergieva, Raju Prasad Srivastava, Bidyapati Jha, Hari Prasad Lamichhane, Gisup Nikha Prasiko, Rashmi Singh, Anup Kumar, Payal Raina, Rajanigandha Tudu, Praveer K.S. Munda, Ion Christian Chiricuta, Ekkasit Tharavichitkul, Razvan M. Galalae, N.E. Kuzmina, N.M. Rostovtsev, V.G. Polyakov, Seema Gupta, Arunima Ghosh, Shraddha Srivastava, Navin Singh

First published in London, United Kingdom, 2022 by IntechOpen
IntechOpen is the global imprint of INTECHOPEN LIMITED, registered in England and Wales, registration number: 11086078, 5 Princes Gate Court, London, SW7 2QJ, United Kingdom
Printed in Croatia

British Library Cataloguing-in-Publication Data
A catalogue record for this book is available from the British Library

Additional hard and PDF copies can be obtained from orders@intechopen.com

Radiation Oncology
Edited by Badruddeen, Usama Ahmad, Mohd Aftab Siddiqui and Juber Akhtar
p. cm.
Print ISBN 978-1-80355-018-3
Online ISBN 978-1-80355-019-0
eBook (PDF) ISBN 978-1-80355-020-6

For EU product safety concerns:
IN TECH d.o.o., Prolaz Marije Krucifikse Kozulić 3, 51000 Rijeka, Croatia, info@intechopen.com or visit our website at intechopen.com.

Meet the editors

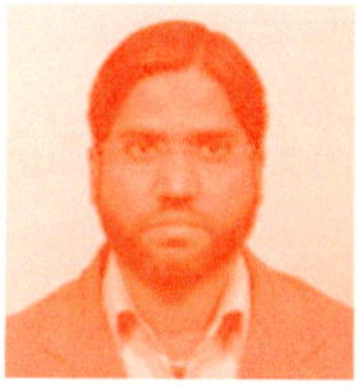

Dr. Badruddeen obtained both a B.Pharm and M.Pharm from Hamdard University, Delhi. He obtained a Ph.D. in Pharmacology from Integral University, Lucknow, in 2014. He qualified for GATE in 2005 & 2006. He has expertise in cardiovascular, neurodegenerative, and endocrine diseases. Dr. Badruddeen has experience in conducting research on the safety, toxicity, and clinical efficacy of herbal and allopathic drugs. He has many original articles in reputed journals to his credit. Dr. Badruddeen is also an editorial board member for several journals. He has supervised a dozen research scholars and is a member of The Indian Science Congress Association, member secretary of the Institutional Animal Ethics Committee (IAEC), coordinator of the Adverse Drug Monitoring Center (AMC), and in charge, of animal house facility, Integral University.

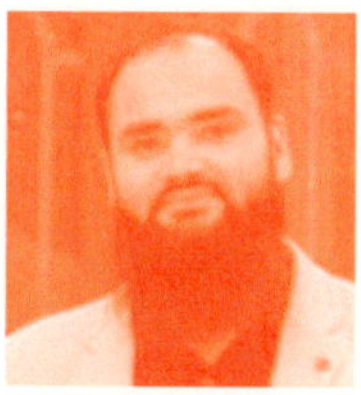

Dr. Usama Ahmad holds a specialization in Pharmaceutics from Amity University, Lucknow, India. He received his Ph.D. from Integral University, Lucknow, India, with his work titled 'Development and evaluation of silymarin nanoformulation for hepatic carcinoma'. Currently, he is an Assistant Professor of Pharmaceutics, at the Faculty of Pharmacy, Integral University. He has been teaching PharmD, BPharm, and MPharm students and conducting research in the novel drug delivery domain. From 2013 to 2014 he worked on a research project funded by SERB-DST, Government of India. He has a rich publication record with more than twenty-four original journal articles, two edited books, four book chapters, and several scientific articles to his credit. He is a member of the American Association for Cancer Research, the International Association for the Study of Lung Cancer, and the British Society for Nanomedicine. Dr. Ahmad's research focus is on the development of nanoformulations to facilitate the delivery of drugs.

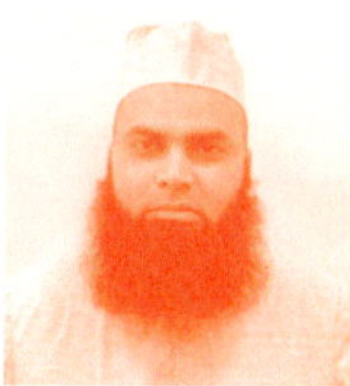

Dr. Juber Akhtar obtained a BPharm from Jamia Hamdard University, New Delhi, in 2005, MPharm from Manipal University, Karnataka, in 2007, and Ph.D. from Integral University, Lucknow, in 2014. He is currently an associate professor at Integral University. From 2014 to 2016, Dr. Akhtar was head of the Faculty of Pharmacy, Integral University. He also served as chairman cum biological scientist for Institutional Animal Ethics Committee (IAEC) from October 2015 to May 2017. He has experience teaching abroad and was previously a professor at Buraydah College of Pharmacy and Dentistry, Kingdom of Saudi Arabia (KSA). Dr. Akhtar has more than eighty publications in reputed journals and is an editorial board member for many esteemed journals. He has supervised a dozen Ph.D. and MPharm students in research projects. Dr. Akhtar's areas of research interest include the development of nanoparticulate drug delivery systems.

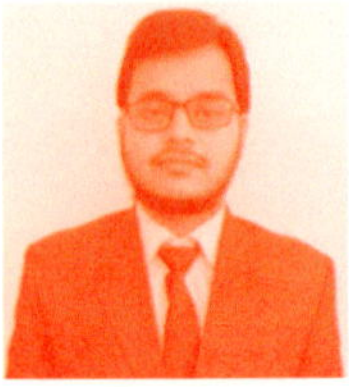

Dr. Mohd Aftab Siddiqui is an assistant professor in the Faculty of Pharmacy, Integral University, Lucknow, India, where he obtained a Ph.D. in Pharmacology in 2020. He also obtained a BPharm and MPharm from the same university in 2013 and 2015, respectively. His area of research is the pharmacological screening of herbal drugs/natural products in liver cancer and cardiac diseases. He is a member of many professional bodies and has guided many MPharm and PharmD research projects. Dr. Siddiqui has many national and international publications and one German patent to his credit.

Contents

Preface

There are several therapeutic methods for cancer treatment, including surgery, systemic therapy, hormonotherapy, and radiation therapy. The therapeutic application of radiation has developed significantly over the past century. Radiation therapy is employed supplementary to surgery or systematic therapy. It is also used as a single treatment procedure. Radiation therapy utilizes high-energy X-rays, protons, electrons, or other particles to kill tumor cells.

This book discusses radiation techniques such as brachytherapy, external radiation, and photodynamic therapy. In the first stage, localized tumours are generally treated by brachytherapy. Brachytherapy is a form of internal radiation therapy for cancer management where a radioactive source is placed in or close to a tumor to destroy its cells. This treatment is used for breast cancer, optic nerve glioma, and cervical cancer. Ultrasound-guided brachytherapy for cervical cancer is also discussed. External radiation is used for lung, breast, head and neck, and abdomen cancers. Photodynamic therapy is used for retroperitoneal tumors in children. It also appreciably increases the survival rate of patients with retroperitoneal tumors. The book also discusses dosimetry audits, which ensure that the accurate therapeutic dose is delivered to patients undergoing radiotherapy.

This book is a useful resource for students, researchers, clinical practitioners, academicians, and other interested readers.

Dr. Badruddeen
Associate Professor,
Faculty of Pharmacy,
Integral University,
Lucknow, India

Usama Ahmad, Juber Akhtar and Mohd Aftab Siddiqui
Integral University,
Lucknow, India

Section 1

Radiation Therapy

Chapter 1

Modern Radiotherapy Techniques for Breast Cancer Treatment

Raju Prasad Srivastava, Bidyapati Jha,
Hari Prasad Lamichhane and GisupNikha Prasiko

Abstract

There are many radiotherapy techniques used to treat breast cancer. Each techniques have their own limitations. The treatment techniques are valid depending on the facilities available to the department. The patient could be treated any technique as the expert knowledge to the center. This chapter will explain about the techniques used in current practice of breast cancer treatment. It will be explained why one technique procedure is better than others. The dose prescription and protocol will be not discussed. It depends on the department policy and facilities. The chapter will be the practical purpose that readers can use straight.

Keywords: intensity modulated radiotherapy, field in field, three-dimensional conformal radiation therapy, VMAT, brachytherapy, SBRT, deep inspiration breath hold

1. Introduction

Breast cancer is the second common type of cancer worldwide after lung cancer and it is the most frequent cancer in the women [1, 2]. As the report, lung cancer is the first common cancer. Breast cancer alone accounts for 29% of all new cancers among women in 2014 [3] and it is the second cause of cancer death in women both in Europe and in the USA [2, 3].

Therapeutic application of radiation has developed significantly over the past century. The development is momentous. It began with brachytherapy and even now continuing in parallel to the external beam radiation techniques. Gradually the use of fascinating advanced external beam radiation techniques is getting a base standard.

There are several therapeutic methods for breast cancer treatment, such as, surgery, systemic therapy, hormonotherapy, and radiation therapy (RT). Radiation therapy is utilized supplementarily to surgery and/or systematic therapy. It is also used as a single treatment procedure. Breast cancer radiation therapy utilizes high-energy X-rays, protons, electrons, or other particles to kill tumor cells. Radiation therapy for breast cancer can be delivered in two techniques i.e., Brachytherapy and External radiation.

2. Brachytherapy

The primary stage localized tumors are treated by brachytherapy. Brachytherapy is a form of internal radiation therapy for cancer treatment where a potted radioactive source is positioned in or near a tumor to demolish tumor cells. The early stage localized tumors are used to treat by brachytherapy. The tumors have not spread (metastasized) to other parts of the body.

Brachytherapy has been in use for most of the twentieth century. In the 1920s, Keynes used interstitial radium needles to implant the entire breast to treat breast cancer [3]. With the advent of megavoltage radiation, external-beam radiation therapy (EBRT) was used to treat the whole breast, with brachytherapy being utilized as a boost for unresected tumors. The high total doses resulted in poor cosmetic results, and therefore, the trend was to perform lumpectomy followed by EBRT and lower doses of brachytherapy [4, 5].

3. External radiation

External radiation therapy is used for lung, breast, head and neck, abdomen etc. cancer treatment. It is an external device provides high energy X-ray radiation from outside body to the localized tumors. It is reliable, comfortable, and minimum side effects depend on which parts of body is being exposed to radiation.

Besides technological hardware and software advances in delivery and planning systems, the fractionation schemes have changed a lot the last decades with recent hypofractionated radiotherapy schemes or emerging partial-breast irradiation protocols. The technical evolution allowed us a successive reduction in the treatment-related complications such as fibrosis and long-term cardiac toxicity. It has shown that the locoregional control rates increased concentrating more on heart and coronary sparing with four-dimensional (4D) breath-hold techniques. Advanced radiotherapy procedures need to be applied in routine clinical care with maximum safety and efficacy. It increases the benefit of locoregional treatment and to decrease the risks of late complications.

3.1 New techniques in external radiation

The treatment of breast cancer by external radiotherapy varies in organization to organization depending on the conveniences and applying treatment protocol. The radiation dose delivery stays complicated to the thoracic wall after complete mastectomy or to the breast conservation surgery. Radiation fields are mostly tangential to include the breast or thoracic wall. The fields are matched to a supraclavicular field in some cases.

3.2 Three-dimensional conformal radiotherapy (3D-CRT)

Three-dimensional conformal radiation therapy (3D CRT) is an advanced technique that includes the use of new imaging technologies computed tomography (CT), magnetic resonance imaging (MRI), positron emission tomography (PET) CT etc.). It generates three-dimensional images of a tumor. 3D CRT permits for a high level of accuracy and the accuracy in the delivery of radiation treatment. The planning target volume (PTV) and organ at risk for three-dimensional conformal radiotherapy (3DCRT) have been defined according to international commission on radiation units & measurements (ICRU) reports 50 and 62 [5, 6]. 3D CRT can use high-energy X-ray beams to be delivered to breast, pelvis head and neck etc. tumors to minimize the dose to the organ at risk.

Treatment plans are independently calculated for each patient. There is various combination such as gantry angles, beam weightage, multi leaf collimator (MLC) positioning, number of fields including field in field (FiF). These are the effective ways to reduce heart dose with 3DCRT in the treatment of breast cancer (**Figure 1**).

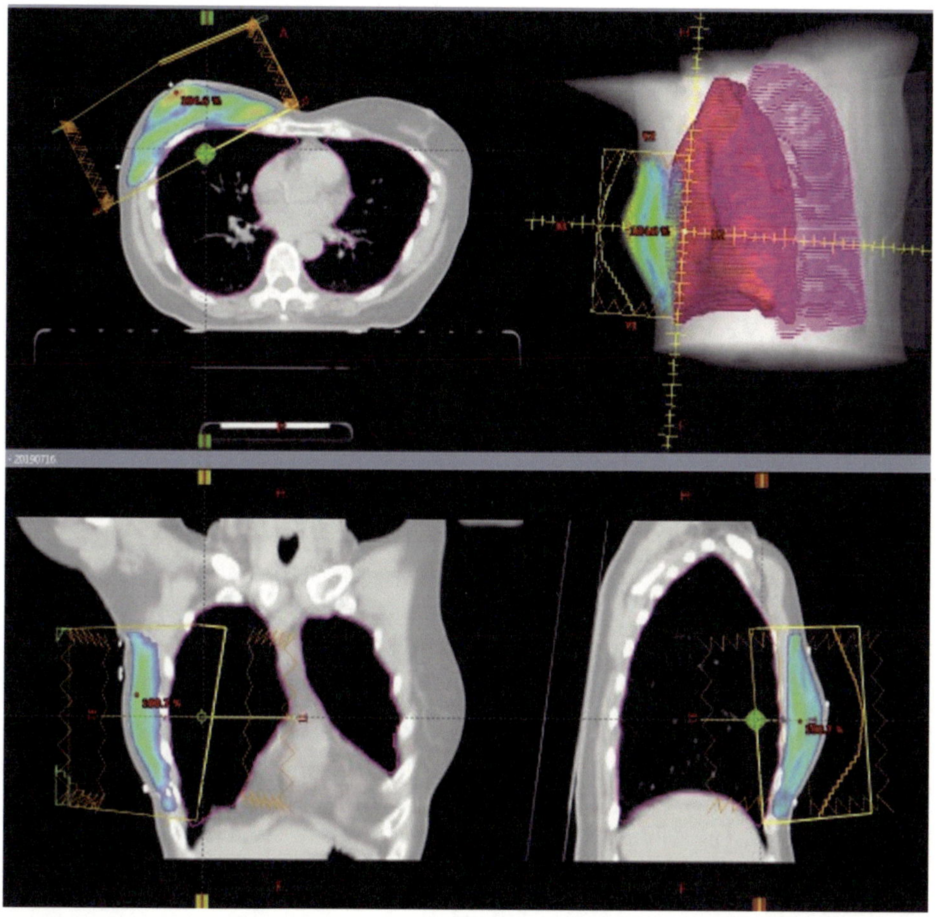

Figure 1.
The figure displays the dose distribution on transversal, coronal, sagittal plane and beams eye view (BEV) for a right-side breast cancer planning using FiF technique. The breast PTV is shown as a blue contour and the colourwash represents 95% of the prescription dose.

3.3 Monoisocentric techniques

The mono isocentric technique reduces the dose in organs at risk such as lung and heart. It also allows the avoidance of the cold and the hot spots. A single isocenter is placed in the junction of tangential and supraclavicular fields. The superior half of the tangential fields and the lower half of the anterior field are half-blocked. The field matching accepted using asymmetric jaws to beam-split along the central axis plane. The treatment delivery needs one time to do set up inside the treatment room to treat tangential and supraclavicular fields. The total treatment delivery time is effectively reduced (**Figure 2**).

3.4 Intensity modulated radiotherapy (IMRT)

Intensity modulated radiation therapy (IMRT) is a modern treatment technique entrenched on delivery of non-uniform fluence. IMRT treatment delivers radiation beams at several different gantry, collimator angles and strengths to provide precise doses to PTV of breast cancer while sparing the dose to organ at risk such as heart, lungs, contra lateral breast and normal tissue. The treatment delivery can be either

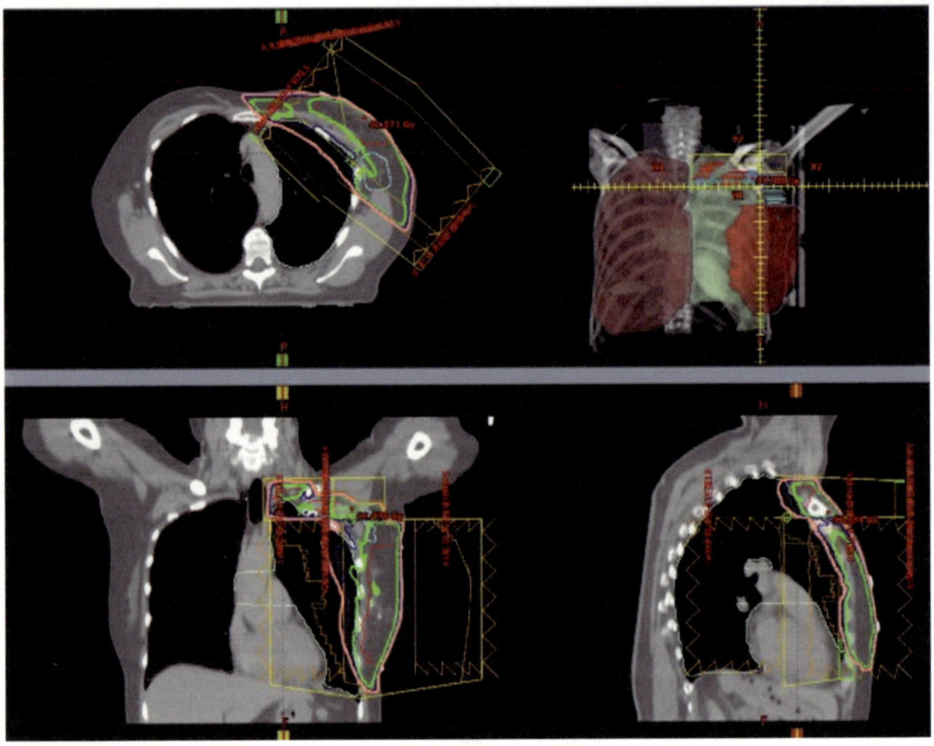

Figure 2.
The figure illustrates the dose distribution on transversal, coronal, sagittal plane and beams eye view (BEV) for left-side breast cancer planning in mono-isocentric technique for irradiation of tangential breast fields and supraclavicular field.

with fixed field or dynamic MLC technique. Dosimetric studies have well recognized advantage of tangent IMRT compared to 2D conventional planning or 3DCRT in providing better PTV coverage and organ at risk (OAR) sparing. Intrafraction motion lowers treatment plans predominantly for treatment of left breast. This motion can be restricted by breath-hold or respiratory gated techniques [7]. The importance of breast IMRT is well recognized. However, the routine clinical application of breast IMRT must be prudently considered (**Figure 3**).

3.5 Volumatic modulated radiotherapy (VMAT)

Traditionally 2-dimensional or 3D conformal radiation techniques often result in large dose inhomogeneity throughout the treatment volumes, inadequate target coverage, or excessive normal tissue doses especially when coverage to the internal mammary nodes is required. Volumetric modulated arc therapy (VMAT) is a novel procedure extension of intensity-modulated radiotherapy (IMRT). An optimized three-dimensional dose distribution may be delivered in rotation of gantry and collimator simultaneously. Breast planning with volumetric modulated arc therapy has been explored mainly for left-sided breast treatments, with the primary committed of decreasing the heart dose and developing target dose homogeneity. VMAT planning technique that produced acceptable target volume coverage, excellent homogeneity throughout the PTV, and tolerable doses to the normal structures (**Figure 4**).

3.6 Stereotactic body radiotherapy (SBRT)

Stereotactic radiation therapy is most frequently used to treat cranial tumor. The radiation therapy in other parts of the body, such as the lung, spine and liver called

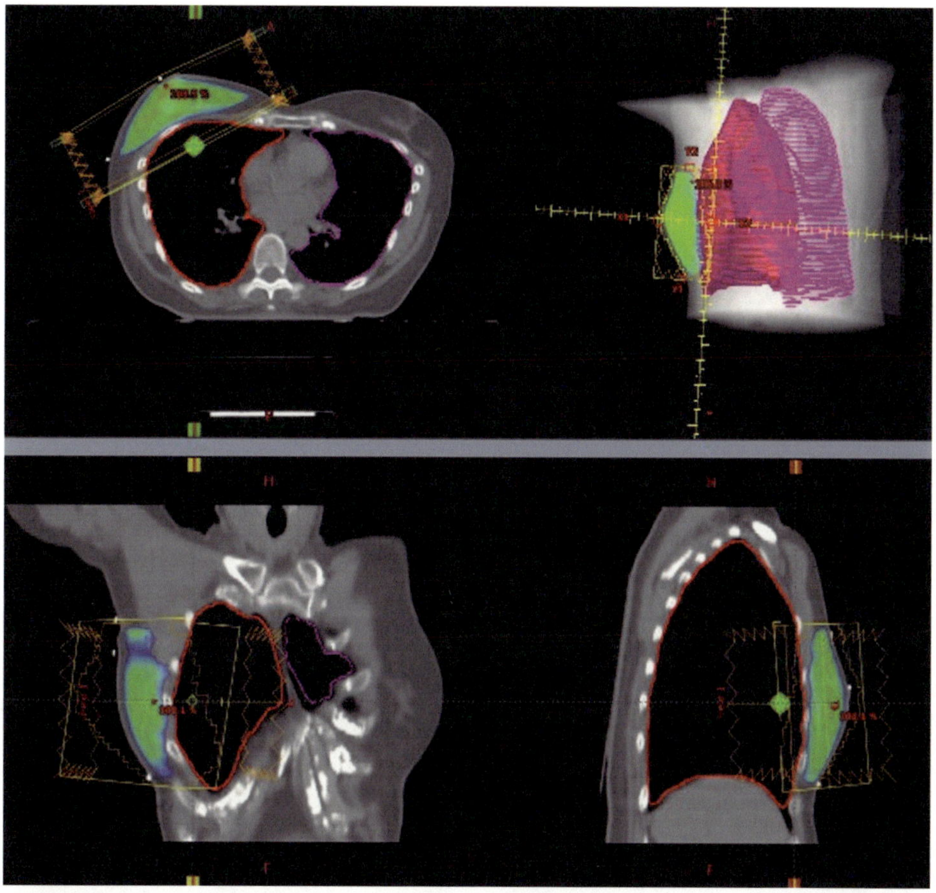

Figure 3.
The figure shows the dose distribution on transversal, coronal, sagittal plane and beams eye view (BEV) for a right-side breast cancer planning using dose dynamic IMRT. The breast PTV is shown as a blue contour and the colourwash represents 95% of the prescription dose.

stereotactic body radiation therapy (SBRT). It delivers a high dose per fraction in a single or multiple fractions. The radiation dose delivers directly to the tumor, sparing nearby healthy tissue. The data of breast SBRT are not established sufficient. It has not validated in a significant prospective study with long term follow up in terms of long-term disease control. Stereotactic body radiation therapy for breast cancer may replace surgery in patients who wish to avoid surgery.

3.7 Deep inspiration breath hold technique

Deep inspiration breath hold (DIBH) is a radiation therapy treatment technique. Patients hold a deep breath throughout while radiation is given. By holding a deep breath in, lungs fill with air and heart will move away from chest wall. The TPS planned and expected delivery doses could be different due to respiratory motion during the treatment delivery. Several research showed that PTV dose heterogeneity increases as respiratory motion grows. The lung and heart doses also change due to respiratory motion. So that a larger margin is suggested from CTV to PTV margin [7]. DIBH technique could help to reduce the dose to heart and lung arising from respiratory motion. Breath-hold technique's dosimetric advantages have been clearly in the literature [8], although the technique is not yet in widespread use.

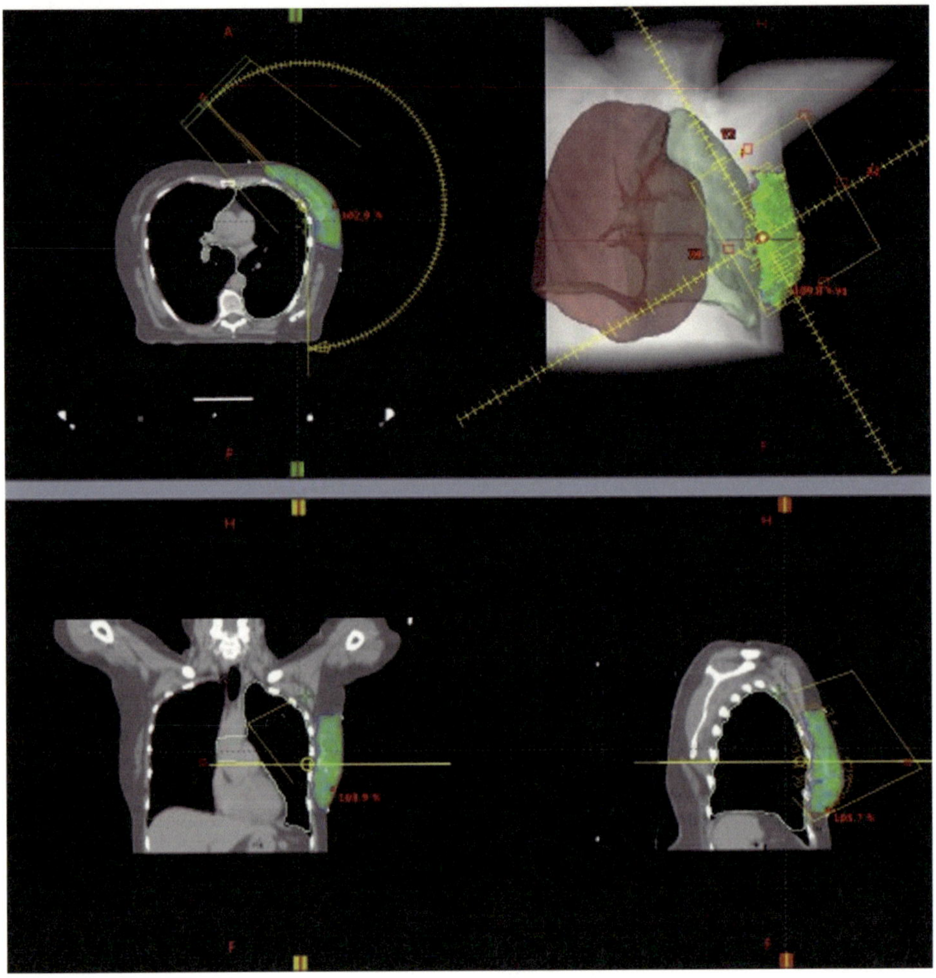

Figure 4.
The dose distribution on transversal, coronal, sagittal plane and beams eye view (BEV) for a left breast cancer planning using VMAT. The breast PTV is shown as a red contour and the colourwash represents 95% of the prescription dose.

3.8 Prone breast irradiation

The supine (face up) position is common for most patients undergoing breast conservation radiation treatment. Prone breast irradiation technique is a special technique to treat breast cancer. The patient placed comfortably on a specially constructed treatment table with a breast board in the prone position (face down) to deliver radiation dose. This technique has become both feasible and reproducible [9] with the help of CT and MRI treatment planning system. The heart may be particularly at risk to late effects of radiation when treatment is given in the supine position for left breast [10] (**Figure 5**).

Recent studies [11, 12] have demonstrated good coverage of PTV and a significant reduction in dose to ipsilateral lung, thyroid, contralateral breast, contralateral lung, and esophagus when compared to supine position. However, prone breast radiation may not be appropriate for all women.

3.9 Proton beam therapy (PBT)

Proton beat therapy (PBT) is a special treatment that can precisely target to PTV and provide high radiation doses to a tumor. The clinical application of proton beam

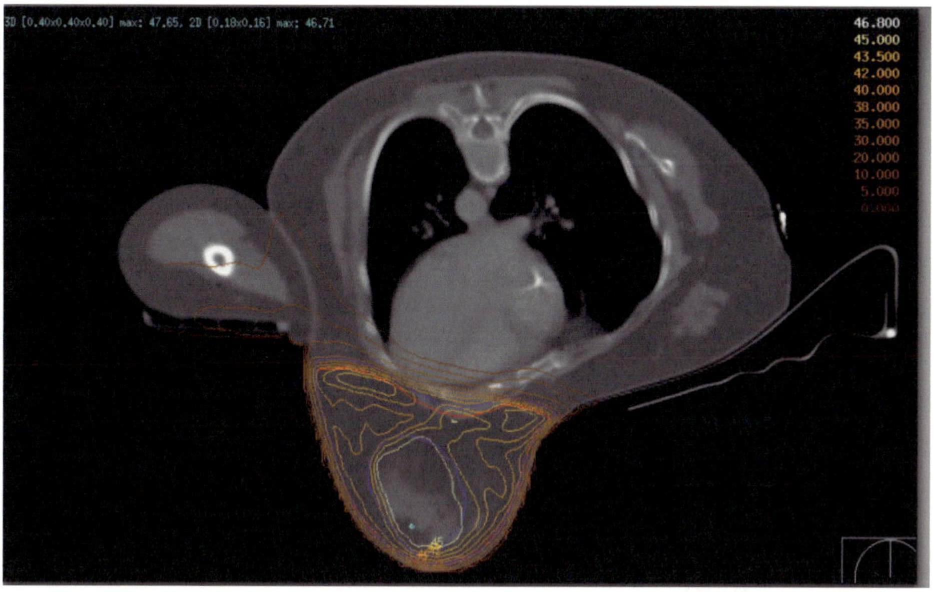

Figure 5.
The dose distribution on transversal beams eye view (BEV) for a left breast cancer planning using VMAT in prone position. The breast PTV is shown as a blue contour and the isodose represents as a color bar.

external radiotherapy has been rising in breast cancer treatment. Bragg peak of proton beam gives the advantage of excellent PTV coverage and reducing damage to neighboring tissue and organs at risk such as the heart and lungs. PBT brings carefully potential to reduce the risk of cardiac events, maintaining the mean heart dose at ≤1 Gy [13].

PBT radiobiological effect rate is higher than (1.1) photons beam. Extensive cost of equipment and maintenance are an important barrier fact to become widespread in clinical use although it has high dosimetric advantage. The current studies [14, 15] showed the great benefit of PBT for breast cancer patients compared to conventional treatment with photon beam.

3.10 Hybrid irradiation

Modern dynamic irradiation techniques by linear accelerators, such as field in Filed (FiF), intensity-modulated radiation therapy (IMRT) and volumetric modulated arc therapy (VMAT), at the time to generate more uniform and conformal dose distributions for the planning target volume (PTV) and less dose to OAR [16, 17]. However, dynamic radiation techniques allow the risk of increased induction of secondary tumors at compliment to larger areas of low-dose exposure and increased monitor units (MU) [18]. To equilibrium the respective benefits of static and dynamic radiation techniques, Mayo et al. [19] have established a composite method combining 3DCRT and IMRT named hybrid intensity-modulated radiation therapy (H-IMRT) (**Figure 6**).

Hybrid is an advanced new technique which uses conventional 3-Dimensional Conformal Radiotherapy (3DCRT) and Intensity Modulated Radiotherapy (IMRT) or Volumetric Modulated Arc Therapy (VMAT). Normally, the ratio of 3DCRT and IMRT or VMAT needs to be determined. The different proportions of 3DCRT and VMAT were used for breast cancer patients to determine the optimal weightage for hybrid technique so that the planning target volume (PTV) coverage improve as well as the dose to the organ at risk (OAR) decline.

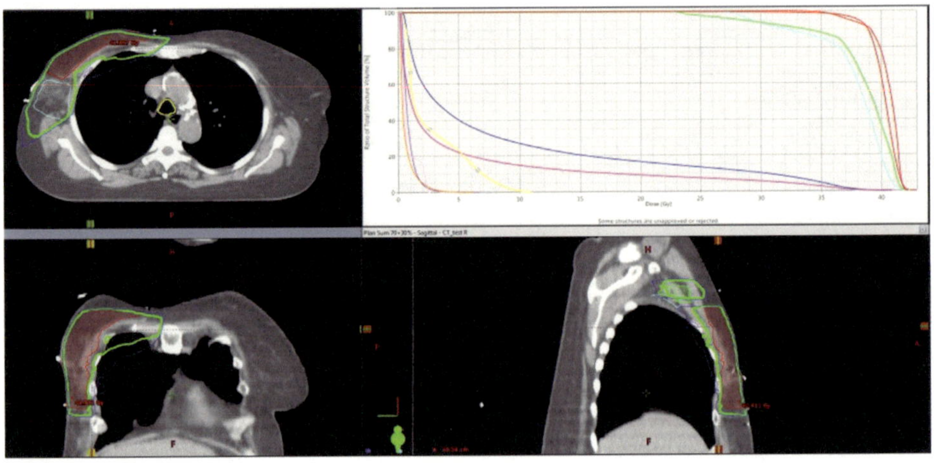

Figure 6.
The figure shows the dose distribution on transversal, DVH, coronal, sagittal planes respectively for 70% 3D FiF plus 30% VMAT (hybrid plane). The green and blue line indicate 95% and 90 isodose line covering PTV (red line).

4. Quality assurance

Patient specific quality assurance is a method for verification of the clinical planned dose before to start the treatment. The planned dose is compared

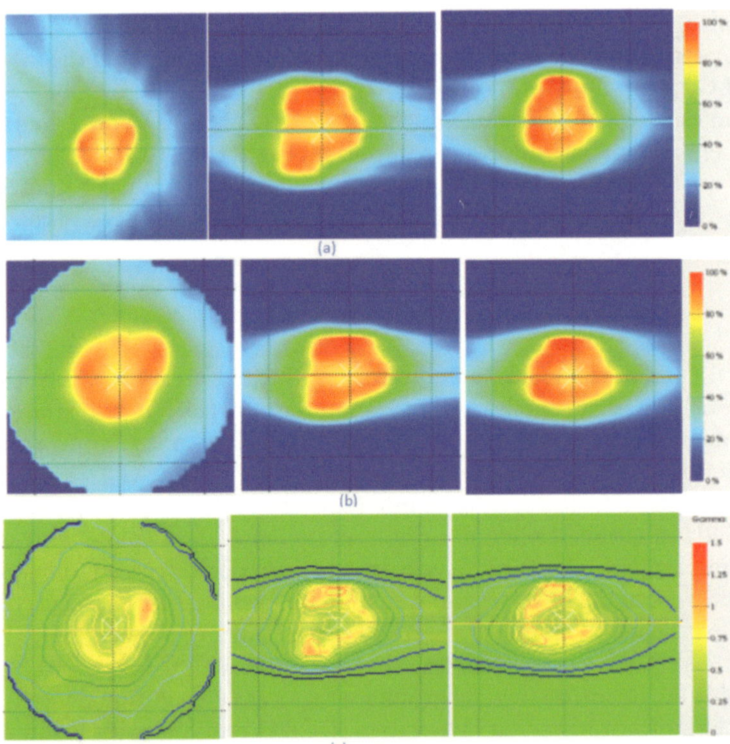

Figure 7.
A screenshot from Octavius 4D measurement analyzed in Verisoft. Showing the result of 3 beams SBRT delivery of lung cases. Panels (a), (b), and (c) show dose map in eclipse, Octavius calculated dose matrices and γ-distribution in transversal, sagittal and coronal plans column wise respectively having 3 beams of SBRT delivery for lung case (figure is taken from [21]).

to delivered dose. The methodology contains various dosimetric tasks that have been performed prior to the treatment of individual patient. Any dose calculation or delivery errors would be revealed. Patient specific QA has benefit to target. The underdose or overdose are harm to the patient. Patient specific QA has been done by film dosimetry, Delta4 phantom [20], Octavius 4D phantom [21], EPID, MapCHECK etc. Each device has their own advantages (**Figure** 7).

Author details

Raju Prasad Srivastava[1,2*], Bidyapati Jha[3,4], Hari Prasad Lamichhane[4] and GisupNikha Prasiko[5]

1 Department of Radiation Oncology, Ghent University Hospital, Corneel Heymanslaan, Ghent, Belgium

2 Centre Hospitalier de Mouscron, Radiothérapie Département, Avenue de Fécamp, Mouscron, Belgium

3 Department of Radiation Oncology, Bhaktapur Cancer Hospital, Dudhpati, Bhaktapur, Nepal

4 Central Department of Physics, Institute of Science & Technology, Tribhuvan 4 University, Kirtipur, Kathmandu, Nepal

5 Nepal Cancer Hospital and Research Center, Harsiddhi, Latitpur, Nepal

*Address all correspondence to: rajupsrivastava@hotmail.com

References

[1] Coleman MP, Quaresma M, Berrino F, Lutz J-M, De Angelis R, Capocaccia R, et al. Cancer survival in five continents: A worldwide population-based study (CONCORD). The Lancet Oncology. 2008;**9**:730-756. DOI: 10.1016/S1470-2045(08)70179-7

[2] Ferlay J, Soerjomataram I, Dikshit R, Eser S, Mathers C, Rebelo M, et al. Cancer incidence and mortality worldwide: Sources, methods and major patterns in GLOBOCAN 2012. International Journal of Cancer. 2015;**136**:E359-E386. DOI: 10.1002/ijc.29210

[3] Siegel R, Ma J, Zou Z, Jemal A. Cancer statistics, 2014. CA: A Cancer Journal for Clinicians. 2014;**64**:9-29. DOI: 10.3322/caac.21208

[4] Keynes G. The treatment of primary carcinoma of the breast with radium. Acta Radiologica. 1929;**10**:393-402. DOI: 10.3109/00016922909132211

[5] Jones D. ICRU report 50—Prescribing, recording and reporting photon beam therapy. Medical Physics. 1994;**21**:833-834. DOI: 10.1118/1.597396

[6] Landberg T, Chavaudra J, Dobbs J, Gerard J-P, Hanks G, Horiot J-C, et al. Report 62. Journal of the International Commission on Radiation Units and Measurements. 1999;**1**:NP. DOI: 10.1093/jicru/os32.1.Report62

[7] Purdy JA. Current ICRU definitions of volumes: Limitations and future directions. Seminars in Radiation Oncology. 2004;**14**:27-40. DOI: 10.1053/j.semradonc.2003.12.002

[8] Bergom C, Currey A, Desai N, Tai A, Strauss JB. Deep inspiration breath hold: Techniques and advantages for cardiac sparing during breast cancer irradiation. Frontiers in Oncology. 2018;**8**:87. DOI: 10.3389/fonc.2018.00087

[9] Grann A, McCormick B, Chabner ES, Gollamudi SV, Schupak KD, Mychalczak BR, et al. Prone breast radiotherapy in early-stage breast cancer: A preliminary analysis. International Journal of Radiation Oncology* Biology* Physics. 2000;**47**:319-325. DOI: 10.1016/S0360-3016(00)00448-X

[10] Taylor CW, Kirby AM. Cardiac side-effects from breast cancer radiotherapy. Clinical Oncology. 2015;**27**:621-629. DOI: 10.1016/j.clon.2015.06.007

[11] Deseyne P, Speleers B, De Neve W, Boute B, Paelinck L, Van Hoof T, et al. Whole breast and regional nodal irradiation in prone versus supine position in left sided breast cancer. Radiation Oncology. 2017;**12**:89. DOI: 10.1186/s13014-017-0828-6

[12] Boute B, De Neve W, Speleers B, Van Greveling A, Monten C, Van Hoof T, et al. Potential benefits of crawl position for prone radiation therapy in breast cancer. Journal of Applied Clinical Medical Physics. 2017;**18**:200-205. DOI: 10.1002/acm2.12118

[13] Verma V, Shah C, Mehta MP. Clinical outcomes and toxicity of proton radiotherapy for breast cancer. Clinical Breast Cancer. 2016;**16**:145-154. DOI: 10.1016/j.clbc.2016.02.006

[14] Braunstein LZ, Cahlon O. Potential morbidity reduction with proton radiation therapy for breast cancer. Seminars in Radiation Oncology. 2018;**28**:138-149. DOI: 10.1016/j.semradonc.2017.11.009

[15] MacDonald SM, Patel SA, Hickey S, Specht M, Isakoff SJ, Gadd M, et al. Proton therapy for breast cancer after mastectomy: Early outcomes of a prospective clinical trial. International Journal of Radiation Oncology* Biology*

Physics. 2013;**86**:484-490. DOI: 10.1016/j.ijrobp.2013.01.038

[16] Dogan N, Cuttino L, Lloyd R, Bump EA, Arthur DW. Optimized dose coverage of regional lymph nodes in breast cancer: The role of intensity-modulated radiotherapy. International Journal of Radiation Oncology* Biology* Physics. 2007;**68**:1238-1250. DOI: 10.1016/j.ijrobp.2007.03.059

[17] Kestin LL, Sharpe MB, Frazier RC, Vicini FA, Yan D, Matter RC, et al. Intensity modulation to improve dose uniformity with tangential breast radiotherapy: Initial clinical experience. International Journal of Radiation Oncology* Biology* Physics. 2000;**48**:1559-1568

[18] Hall EJ. Intensity-modulated radiation therapy, protons, and the risk of second cancers. International Journal of Radiation Oncology* Biology* Physics. 2006;**65**:1-7

[19] Mayo CS, Urie MM, Fitzgerald TJ. Hybrid IMRT plans—Concurrently treating conventional and IMRT beams for improved breast irradiation and reduced planning time. International Journal of Radiation Oncology* Biology* Physics. 2005;**61**:922-932

[20] Srivastava RP, Wagter CD. Clinical experience using Delta 4 phantom for pretreatment patient-specific quality assurance in modern radiotherapy. Journal of Radiotherapy in Practice. 2019;**18**:210-214. DOI: 10.1017/S1460396918000572

[21] Srivastava RP, Basta K, Thevissen K, Junius S, Vandeputte K, Wagter C. Gamma evaluation with octavius 4D phantom for pre-treatment of modern radiotherapy treatment techniques. International Journal of Nuclear Medicine and Radioactive Substances. 2019;**2**(2):000117

Chapter 2

Photodynamic Therapy in Complex Therapy of Retroperitoneal Tumors in Children

N.M. Rostovtsev, V.G. Polyakov and N.E. Kuzmina

Abstract

During the period from 2009 to 2021, 93 patients aged 0–11 years (48 boys and 45 girls) with retroperitoneal tumors were treated. There were 66 patients with nephroblastoma and 27 patients with adrenal neuroblastoma among them. As per treatment strategies, the patients were separated into two groups: the control group and the study group. The control group (comparison) received therapy according to the protocols, whereas the study group consisted of patients who received photodynamic therapy (PDT) in addition to the standard treatment. The control group consists of 47 patients with retroperitoneal tumors, including 35 patients with nephroblastoma and 12 patients with adrenal neuroblastoma. The study group included 46 children: 31 patients with nephroblastoma and 15 patients with adrenal neuroblastoma. The 5-year survival rate in the control group was 74.5%, and it was 91.3% in the study group ($p = 0.030$). Recurrent tumors developed in 14.9% of the patients in the control group, while in the study group, relapse occurred in 8.7% of the patients ($p = 0.357$). The PDT used in this study for treatment of retroperitoneal tumors improves the results of surgical treatment. It also appreciably increases the survival rate of patients with retroperitoneal tumors. Overall, PDT is a hopeful antitumor approach and can be effectively used in the complex therapy of retroperitoneal tumors in children.

Keywords: children, photodynamic therapy, nephroblastoma, neuroblastoma, radachlorin

1. Introduction

The problems of pediatric oncology are quite urgent, since malignant neoplasms are leading in the structure of child mortality worldwide, second only to external causes. The incidence of cancer cases is estimated by the World Health Organization (WHO) as about 100 per million children. These are rare diseases among the pediatric population, ranging from 0.5 to 4.6% of all cancers [1, 2].

Neuroblastoma (NB) and nephroblastoma, or Wilms' tumor (WT), are the two most common extracranial solid tumors in childhood [3, 4]. Both tumors are most often located in the retroperitoneal space, develop from embryonic cells, and in most cases are diagnosed in children younger than 5 years [4]. NB is an embryonic malignant tumor arising from the ganglia of the borderline sympathetic trunk and chromaffin tissue. The prevalence of NB is estimated as 1 case per 7000–10,000 live births, it accounts for 6–10% of all malignancies in children [5, 6]. The most common localizations of this tumor are adrenal glands (40%) and retroperitoneal space (25%), less often NB develops in the posterior mediastinum (15%), in the neck (5%) and pelvis minor (5%). The prevalence of WT, which is the most common kidney tumor in childhood, is 1 case per 10,000 children under the age of 15 [7]. About 10% of cases of the disease are associated with the presence in patients of such congenital syndromes as WAGR syndrome, Beckwith-Wiedemann syndrome, Denys-Drash syndrome, and hemihypertrophy [8]. From the point of view of embryogenesis, WT is a solid malignant tumor consisting of derivatives of nephrogenic tissue at different degrees of differentiation. These tumors may contain not only a variety of tissue elements present in a normal kidney, but also skeletal muscles, cartilages, mucosal and stratified squamous epithelium. In typical cases, WT is a large solid growth, often with areas of necrosis, hemorrhages, and cysts. However, in about 7% of cases, WT is a multifocal growth. The tumor can spread to the pelvis and ureter, causing obstruction of the urinary tract. In addition, it can invade the intrarenal blood and lymph vessels, penetrate the renal capsule, and grow into the paranephric and other adjacent tissues, spread from the renal vein into the inferior vena cava [4].

2. Clinical manifestations

It should be noted that retroperitoneal tumor in children is primarily not clinically manifested and has no specificity during a long period of time. The primary tumor symptom complex is a variety of pathological manifestations caused by the influence of the tumor process on metabolism, immunity, and functional activity of the regulatory systems of the body. The most common symptoms are physical inactivity, lack of appetite, weight loss, lethargy, asthenia, rapid fatigability, moodiness, anemia, low-grade fever, and abdominal pain. The syndrome of minor signs of a tumor is present in most patients, but usually neither parents nor doctors attach significant importance to it. Usually, the first clinical manifestation is a palpable tumor in the abdomen, which is found accidentally. The tumor is smooth, sometimes coarse-grained, dense, painless, and moderately mobile. Macrohematuria occurs in less than 1/4 of patients and is considered a manifestation of tumor invasion into the renal pelvis system. Arterial hypertension is often observed [9].

Surgical treatment of both tumors is mandatory in antitumor therapy. In accordance with the recommendations of the SIOP (International Society of Pediatric Oncology) protocol used in European countries, chemotherapy is performed within 4 weeks before surgery in order to reduce the risk of intraoperative tumor rupture [10, 11].

Successful treatment of solid tumors involves early diagnosis, radical removal of the tumor with an extensive operative exploration of abdominal organs and regional lymph nodes, as well as neoadjuvant and adjuvant chemotherapy. The use of ablastic methods in the surgical treatment of tumors, which include photodynamic therapy (PDT), is becoming extremely important.

PDT is a treatment method based on the use of photosensitive substances, i.e., photosensitizers (FS) and light of a certain wavelength. FS selectively accumulates in the tumor tissue, then the affected tissues are illuminated with the light generated by special surgical laser units. As a result of subsequent cellular photochemical reactions, reactive oxygen species are released destroying pathological cells, causing nutrition disorders, leading to tumor apoptosis due to the damage to its micro-vessels. The antitumor effects of PDT in vivo result from three interrelated mechanisms, namely direct cytotoxic effects on tumor cells, damage to the tumor vascular network, and induction of a strong inflammatory reaction that can result in the development of a systemic immune response [12–15]. The established presence of an immunological component of photodynamic effect indicates the prospects of combining PDT and immunotherapy methods to improve the results of cancer treatment [16].

The use of photodynamic therapy in the treatment of oncological diseases has begun relatively recently. To date, the vast majority of works devoted to the use of PDT are studies carried out in the adult population, their purpose is to clarify the therapeutic effectiveness of PDT, identify priority FS and the scope of their application [17, 18].

However, the problem has been little studied in pediatric population, since it is associated with certain difficulties caused by limited technical capabilities and lack of application experience. Despite the great interest of researchers in this method, there are few data on the use of PDT in pediatric patients. There are only some works indicating the high efficiency of PDT application in pediatric dentistry, dermatology, and ophthalmology [19–22].

Nevertheless, the anatomical and physiological features of childhood require the development of specific therapeutic techniques: namely schemes and modes of use, taking into account the age and severity of the disease. We have not found data about the methodology and optimal modes of PDT, as well as the use of Radachlorine as FS for the treatment of solid tumors and the prevention of intra-operative metastasis in children in the literature review. This made it necessary to further study the possibilities of PDT in the treatment of solid tumors in children and determine the purpose and objectives of this study. Taking into account the data obtained during the preclinical study [23], we are to prove the effectiveness of PDT using Radachlorine photosensitizer aiming at increasing the clinical efficiency (5-year survival rate) of treatment of children with solid retroperitoneal tumors.

3. Materials and methods

The study was performed in the surgical department and Oncologic Hematology Center for Children and Adolescents named after Professor V.I. Gerain of the State Budgetary Healthcare Institution "Chelyabinsk Regional Children's Clinical Hospital."

The studied group consisted of 93 patients with retroperitoneal tumors (48 boys and 45 girls), 66 patients with nephroblastoma, 27 patients with adrenal neuro-blastoma. Taking into account the performed therapy, the patients were divided into two groups: the comparison group and the study group. The comparison group (control) received therapy according to the protocols SIOP 93, SIOP 2001, NB2004. The study group consisted of patients who received photodynamic therapy in addition to the standard treatment.

The comparison group included 47 patients with retroperitoneal tumors, including 35 patients with nephroblastoma and 12 patients with adrenal neuroblastoma. The study group included 46 children: 31 patients with nephroblastoma and 15 patients with adrenal neuroblastoma. The distribution of patients into treatment groups depending on the type of tumor is shown in **Table 1**.

The patients of the clinical groups were divided into age subgroups according to the age periodization according to A.V. Mazurin, I. M. Vorontsov [24]. **Table 2** shows the distribution of patients by age.

Depending on the gender, the patients of the studied groups were distributed in the following way as presented in **Table 3**.

Clinical groups (n = 93)	Tumor	
	nephroblastoma	neuroblastoma
Comparison group (n = 47)	35	12
Study group (n = 46)	31	15

Table 1.
Distribution of patients into clinical groups depending on the type of tumor.

Clinical groups (n = 93)	Age groups		
	0–3 years	4–6 years	7–12 years
Comparison Group (n = 47)	31	14	2
Study group (n = 46)	31	10	5
Total (n = 93)	62	24	7

Table 2.
Distribution of patients in clinical groups by age.

Clinical groups	boys	girls
Comparison Group (n = 47)	25	22
Study group (n = 46)	23	23
Total (n = 93)	48	45

Table 3.
Distribution of patients into clinical groups depending on gender.

As can be seen from **Table 2**, in both clinical groups, the vast majority of patients are children of early age group from 0 to 3 years, that is, 62 children (66.7%). The next group is preschool-age children from 4 to 6 years, that is, 24 children (25.8%). Retroperitoneal tumors are revealed less frequently in older children, there are only seven patients in the age group older than 7 years (7.5%). The number of boys and girls in the clinical groups of patients is almost the same (**Table 3**): 48 boys (51.6%) and 45 girls (48.4%). The findings received by us do not contradict the literature data [10, 11, 25, 26], according to which retroperitoneal tumors develop more often in children aged 1–3 years, and in 90% of cases, the diagnosis is made before the age of 7. Our study also did not establish gender prevalence in the occurrence of tumor in children. The incidence among boys and girls was the same.

Depending on the therapy to be carried out, the patients were divided into two groups. Patients of the comparison group underwent surgical treatment in combination with chemotherapy and radiation therapy according to the protocol. Patients of the study group received therapy according to the SIOP protocol in combination with PDT.

All children with an identified oncological condition underwent a complex of mandatory diagnostic tests, in accordance with the Clinical Recommendations of the Ministry of Health of the Russian Federation. Patients with retroperitoneal tumors necessarily underwent a physical examination to determine density of the tumor surface, mobility, and size of the growth. Palpation of all accessible groups of peripheral lymph nodes was performed. Blood pressure measurement and neurological status assessment were mandatory.

Laboratory tests included clinical blood analysis, common urine analysis, biochemical blood analysis (electrolytes, whole protein, liver samples, creatinine, urea, lactate dehydrogenase, alkaline phosphatase) and a study for tumor markers of NB catecholamines in urine and serum, NSE (to exclude NB).

Studies of molecular biological markers (N-MYC oncogene amplification and 1p deletion) and histological examination were carried out, and histomorphologic diagnosis in all patients with WT and NB was made. Taking into account the data obtained, the tumor process was staged according to SIOP and NWTS.

Instrumental methods of examination included ultrasound of the abdominal cavity organs and retroperitoneal space with blood flow mapping, CT of the abdominal cavity organs and retroperitoneal space with intravenous contrast, MRI of the abdominal cavity and retroperitoneal space with and without contrast enhancement. If necessary, angiography and a radioisotope study of the kidneys were performed to assess kidney function. Compulsory examinations were electrocardiography and echocardiography.

Special attention was paid to safety and ethical issues of the study.

The study was approved by the local Ethics Committee of GBUZ CHODKB—Protocol No. 17 of 20.03.2015. The sampling of patients was carried out on a voluntary basis. The clinical trial was conducted in accordance with the scientific and moral principles set out in the Helsinki Declaration of the World Medical Association and reflected in OST 42-511-99 "Rules for Conducting Qualitative Clinical Trials in the Russian Federation," ICH GCP rules and current regulatory requirements. All patients were provided with written information about the drug prior to the study. Legal representatives and patients were informed in detail by the doctor who conducted the study about the procedure of introducing a photosensitizer. Before starting the study, the parents signed an informed consent form confirming their voluntary participation.

The inclusion criteria in the study on the effectiveness of PDT in retroperitoneal tumors in children were:

1. a diagnosed malignancy of the retroperitoneal space as an initial condition;

2. guaranteed voluntary continuous follow-up for 60 months (5 years) after surgical intervention and PDT;

3. association between the confirmed tumor and death, as well as the established cause of death;

4. availability of complete information in medical documentation, including case history, laboratory data, diagnostic tests.

Based on the results of a comprehensive examination, an "Individual Case Record" was filled in for each patient, including a complete anamnesis, laboratory data, and diagnostic studies.

An assessment was carried out in both groups of patients after PDT and complex treatment within two months. The effectiveness of therapy was evaluated according to standard criteria (WHO), taking into account the dynamics of surgical treatment, tumor recurrence, as well as the patient's condition. Later, postoperative follow-up was carried out on an outpatient basis for 5 years, every 6 months (10 visits). The tumor was monitored, dynamic data control of laboratory findings, ultrasound, and CT were carried out.

To assess the effectiveness of PDT, the operational characteristics of the test were used in accordance with the principles of evidence-based medicine. Criteria for the effectiveness of the conducted PDT:

- full effect—complete disappearance of all manifestations of the disease, the established complete absence of local recurrence of the tumor according to palpation, visual signs, as well as special diagnostic tests;

- local relapse—occurrence of a local relapse within 6 months following surgery;

- without effect—continued tumor growth according to additional research methods;

- partial effect—absence of a tumor, but presence of enlarged lymph nodes, confirmed at two months post-intervention.

The safety of the participants was ensured:

- no unpleasant sensations from PDT, the procedure being performed under anesthesia intraoperatively;

- protective glasses with a light filter used by a doctor and a patient during laser exposure;

- rapid elimination of Radachlorine from the blood and mucous membranes (high contrast index excludes damage to healthy organs and tissues);

- selective accumulation of Radachlorine in the tumor, absence of mutagenic action on the DNA of normal cells.

There were no valid data on adverse medical consequences published.

Spectral fluorescence examination of patients was carried out before the injection of Radachlorine, every hour after the injection of Radachlorine and after the end of the PDT procedure. The accumulation of photosensitizer in the tumor was measured using a laser electron spectral device LESA-01-Biospec. During the measurement, the spectrum was determined by analyzing its shape and amplitude of the signal, the integral intensity of Radachlorine fluorescence at various sites of the tumor and adjacent tissues, and the fluorescent boundaries of the tumor. Also, the intensity of fluorescence of the normal skin of the hands and face and oral mucosa of patients was evaluated. The ratio between the values of fluorescence intensity in the tumor and normal tissue, which characterized the selectivity of accumulation in the tumor tissue, was determined.

PDT with Radachlorine was performed intraoperatively after removal of the tumor by means of a high-intensity laser "Lakhta Milon" (Russia), using laser illumination in the range of 0.1–0.8 W/cm^2. Depending on the depth of infiltrating tumor growth, various doses of light energy were used—from 150 to 400 J/cm^2, wavelength 650–670 nm, adjusted during an experimental study [23]. The photosensitizer was administered intravenously, at the rate of 0.6–0.8 mg/kg 2–3 hours prior to illumination. The duration of illumination depended on the size of the tumor and averaged 20 minutes.

Statistical data processing was carried out using IBM SPSS Statistics 19 package. The analysis of qualitative characteristics in the studied groups was done by means of construction of cross-tabulation tables and calculation of significance by χ^2-Pirson criterion. The differences were considered statistically significant for p values <0.05, which corresponded to 95% probability of an accurate prediction. To analyze the data of overall 5-year survival and relapse-free survival Kaplan-Meier curves were constructed calculating average survival time, its standard error, and 95% significance interval. A long-range criterion was applied to identify statistical differences in the survival curves. The differences were considered statistically significant for p values <0.05.

4. Results

We could not find information on the use of photodynamic therapy in children in the treatment of retroperitoneal tumors in the available literature sources. General and relapse-free survival of patients in the studied clinical groups was analyzed by the Kaplan-Meier method to assess the effectiveness of treatment results, regarding the percentage of patients who survived after the use of photodynamic therapy. The duration of observation time was from the intraoperative photodynamic therapy to the end of a 5-year follow-up. Based on the data obtained, the mean values of the survival time before the onset of death and mean values before the onset of relapse in patients of the control and study groups were obtained, as shown in **Tables 4** and **6**. The mean time free from any outcome (death, relapse) is a certain number of months, **Tables 5** and 7. The tables also present standard error (SE) and 95% confidence interval (95% CI) values for the mean time value.

A graphical presentation of the Kaplan-Meier method was the curves of the overall 5-year and relapse-free survival, as shown in **Figures 1** and **2**. The ordinate axis shows the probability of outcome occurrence, and the abscissa axis shows time (months).

Clinical groups (n = 93)	Five-year Survival rate (%)	Mortality rate (cases)	Mortality rate (%)
Comparison Group (n = 46)	74.5	12	25.5
Study group (n = 47)	91.3	4	8.7

P = 0.030.

Table 4.
Percentage of cases of fatal outcome in patients with tumor, depending on the treatment method.

Clinical groups	Mean values			
	Estimate	St. error	95% confidence interval	
			Lower range limit	Upper range limit
Comparison group	47.404	3.197	41.138	53.671
Study group	56.022	1.927	52.257	59.786

p = 0.030.

Table 5.
Mean value of survival time before fatal outcome in the studied groups of patients.

Clinical groups (n = 93)	Five-year (%) relapse-free survival rate	Relapses (cases)	Relapses (%)
Comparison Group (n = 46)	85.1	7	14.9
Study group (n = 47)	91.3	4	8.7

p = 0.357.

Table 6.
Percentage of cases of relapse in patients, depending on the treatment method.

Clinical groups	Mean values[a]			
	Estimate	St. error	95% confidence interval	
			Lower range limit	Upper range limit
Comparison group	52.213	2.734	46.855	57.571
Study group	55.477	2.169	51.227	59.728

p = 0.357.

Table 7.
Mean survival time prior to relapse.

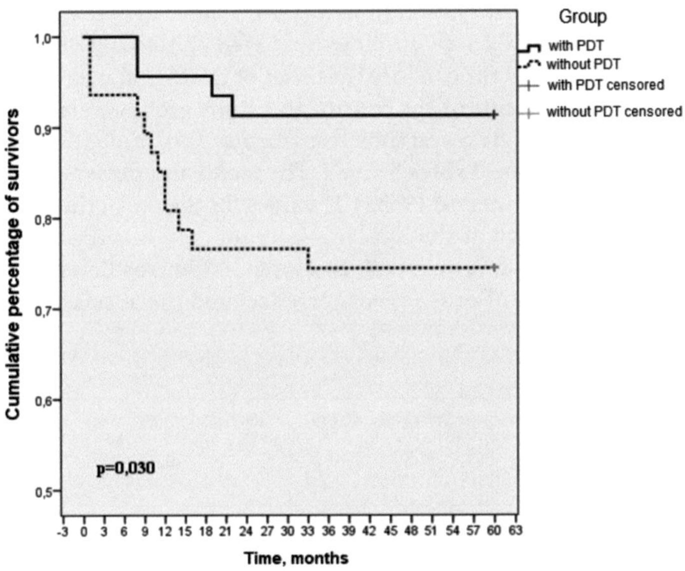

Figure 1.
Overall 5-year survival rate of studied patients.

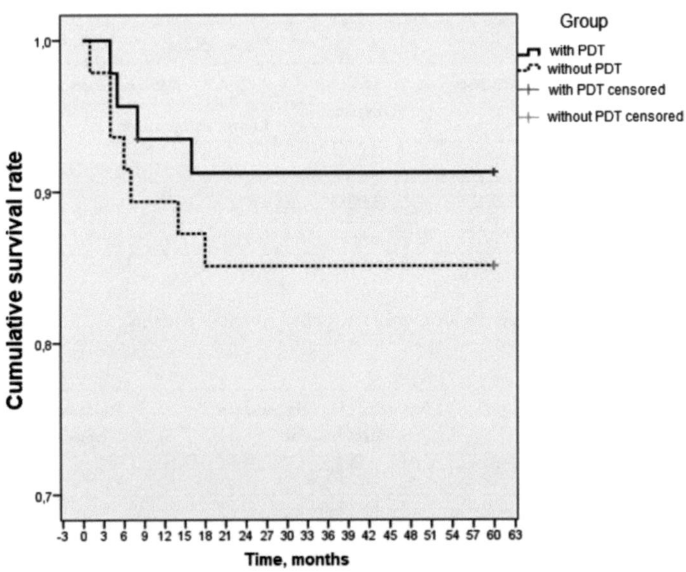

Figure 2.
Comparison of relapse-free survival in studied patients.

5. Discussion

As previously reported, we were able to find only a few studies on the use of PDT in children in dental, dermatological, and ophthalmological practice in literature [19–22]. Reports on the use of PDT in the treatment of retroperitoneal tumors in children could not be found. In our study, we relied on the results of a preliminary trial, during which the scheme and mode of PDT were developed [23]. Radachlorine (FS of the second generation) was used as FS, which has a greater selectivity of accumulation (in comparison with FS of the first generation), which provides a greater depth of damage to tumor tissue due to shifts of absorption maxima to a longer wavelength spectrum (650–670 nm), intact surrounding tissues during illumination and low skin phototoxicity. A good clinical efficacy of PDT with Radachlorine as FS in the treatment of tumors of different localization has been demonstrated in the publications of a number of authors. Moreover, different forms of drug formulation make it possible for both local, including intra-focal, and systemic administration of Radachlorine.

In the work of Sukhova T.E. [27], the response of basal cell skin cancer in its various clinical forms, stages, histological types, course of the disease, and tumor localization to PDT with intra-focal administration of Radachlorine and Photoditazine was studied. The study included 74 patients with primary and recurrent basal cell carcinoma of the skin of stage I–II. The patients of group I (n = 45) were injected with Radachlorine (0.5–1 ml / 1 cm^2 of the tumor surface), patients in group II (n = 34) had Photoditazine (0.3–0.5 ml/1 cm^2 of the tumor surface). The light dose was 300 J/cm^2, the illumination wavelength was 662 ± 3 nm for all patients. As a result of the therapy, a complete regression of basal cell skin cancer was established in 43 patients from group I (95.5%) and in 31 from group II (91.2%). At the same time, PDT with Radachlorine FS significantly improved the results of treatment of the ulcerative form of tumor compared with PDT using Photoditazine FS (92.8% vs. 77.8%, respectively, $p < 0.05$).

Filonenko E.V. et al. [28] used Radachlorine in the treatment of precancerous and tumor diseases of the cervix in 30 patients. Radachlorine was administered once by a 30-minute intravenous infusion at a dose of 1.0 mg/kg body weight 3 hours before illumination (wavelength 662 nm, energy density 300–350 J/cm^2). A good clinical result was achieved in 26 patients (86.7%), it was assessed as complete regression of the tumor, in 4 (13.3%)—as partial regression. It is important that during and after the treatment, there were no adverse reactions to the administration of Radachlorine and PDT.

Vashakmadze L.A. et al. [29] reported on the intraoperative use of Radachlorine in patients with a high risk of local tumor recurrence after surgical treatment. The study included 17 patients with morphologically confirmed operable primary or recurrent retroperitoneal tumor. Intraoperative photodynamic therapy was performed with Photogem (five patients), Radachlorine (seven patients), and Photoditazine (five patients). In nine cases, the tumors had the structure of liposarcoma, in 4—leiomyosarcoma, in 2—gastrointestinal stromal tumor, in 1—neurogenic tumor, in 1—hemangiopericytoma. Photosensitizers were administered intravenously: Photohem 48 hours before surgery at a dose of 2.5–3.0 mg/kg, Radachlorine and Photoditazine—at doses of 0.7 and 0.7–1.0 mg/kg, respectively 2–3 hours before the resection stage of the operation. The tumor bed was illuminated after a complete tumor removal within intact tissues from one or more positions, depending on the location of tumor foci. The illumination energy density was 30 J/cm^2, the duration of the exposure session depended on the illumination area. The accumulation of photosensitizer in the tumor tissue was assessed after removal of the neoplasm using local fluorescence spectroscopy by means of the diagnostic unit "Spectrum." The researchers observed a relapse of the disease after surgical treatment with intraoperative PDT sessions in six (out of 17) patients within a period of 2–6 months. Three patients (out of six) developed local relapses of the disease 2, 4, and 6 months after the treatment (surgery accompanied by intraoperative PDT). The authors remarked that PDT was performed in patients who developed local relapses of the disease at the stage of testing the technique, choosing the modes and radiation dose. The researchers made conclusions about the safety of photodynamic therapy and the precision of the photosensitizer accumulation used to retroperitoneal sarcoma tissue, which was confirmed by local fluorescence spectroscopy data.

The work of this research group was the most interesting and similar in structure to our study. Like other research groups, we expected a good clinical response associated with the high selectivity of Radachlorine and, consequently, with the high photodynamic activity of the drug. Modern fiber-optic technology facilitates the delivery of light of the desired wavelength and energy flux density to tumors located almost anywhere in the body. Local illumination, together with the protection of sensitive tissues at the edge of the area, allows for specific treatment of the tumor without destroying normal tissues outside the treated area. The combination of surgical treatment with intraoperative PDT was used to increase the efficacy of surgical interventions and reduce the number of local relapses.

Analysis of the data of our study showed that in the group of patients receiving therapy according to the protocol, without the additional use of photodynamic therapy, the number of deaths was 12, therefore the survival rate was 74.5%. In patients of the study group who received photodynamic therapy in addition to the standard therapy, the number of fatal outcomes during the 5-year follow-up period was less and amounted to four cases. The survival rate, respectively, was higher—91.3%. Comparison of 5-year survival curves in the control and study groups according to the nonparametric log-rank criterion showed a significant difference in the groups ($p = 0.030$). At the same time, the average survival time before the onset of death in patients who received photodynamic therapy significantly exceeded the mean survival time in patients who received therapy according to the protocol, without additional use of PDT, i.e., 56 months vs. 47 months, respectively ($p < 0.050$).

There was no statistically significant difference in the analysis of relapse-free survival in patients of clinical groups: in the study group, relapse occurred in 8.7% of patients, in the comparison group—in 14.9% of patients ($p = 0.357$). The mean survival time to relapse in both groups had no significant difference and made up 55 months in patients receiving photodynamic therapy versus 52 months in patients not receiving photodynamic therapy ($p = 0.357$).

Nevertheless, the obtained data regarding relapse-free survival are optimistic. Firstly, preclinical studies have shown the possibility of combining PDT regimens that inhibit primary tumor growth and stimulate antitumor immunity [30–32]. In this case, PDT is a potential method that is due to its immunological mechanisms, can strengthen the control of primary and metastatic tumors, and consequently, facilitate recovery and improve the quality of life in cancer patients. Secondly, the selectivity of photosensitizer accumulation in the tumor can be artificially increased by targeted delivery of the drug to tumor cells. Currently, several techniques to selectively target photosensitizer to the tumor are being developed. Search for transport systems that provide even higher selectivity and precision is described in the world literature [33]. We believe that the method is promising in terms of further research and the accumulation of clinical experience, and the development of exposure modes will allow assessing its effectiveness and impact on the recurrence rate in extra-organ retroperitoneal tumors.

6. Conclusions

The proposed method of complex treatment of retroperitoneal tumors using PDT allows improvement of the results of surgical treatment; it significantly increases the survival rate of patients with retroperitoneal tumors (91.3% vs. 74.5%) ($p < 0.050$). Thus, PDT is a promising antitumor strategy, technically possible, and can be successfully used in the complex therapy of retroperitoneal tumors in children.

Author details

N.M. Rostovtsev[1,2*], V.G. Polyakov[3] and N.E. Kuzmina[1]

1 GBUZ Chelyabinsk Regional Children's Clinical Hospital, Chelyabinsk, Russia

2 FGBOU VO "South Ural State Medical University" of the Ministry of Health of the Russian Federation, Chelyabinsk, Russia

3 FGBU Blokhin National Medical Research Center of Oncology named after N.N. Blokhin, Moscow, Russia

*Address all correspondence to: rostovcevnm@mail.ru

References

[1] Rykov MY, Sevryukov DD, Vilkova AS. Malignant neoplasms in children: Clinical manifestations and diagnosis. Issues of Modern Pediatrics. 2017;**16**(5):370-382

[2] Fathi A, Bahadoram M, Amani F. Epidemiology of childhood cancer in Northwest Iran. Asian Pacific Journal of Cancer Prevention. 2015;**16**:5459-5462

[3] Dickson PV, Sims TL, Streck CJ, et al. Avoiding misdiagnosing neuroblastoma as Wilms tumor. Journal of Pediatric Surgery. 2008;**43**(6):1159-1163

[4] Meyer JS, Harty MP, Khademian Z. Imaging of neuroblastoma and Wilms' tumor. Magnetic Resonance Imaging Clinics of North America. 2002;**10**(2): 275-302

[5] Kim S, Chung DH. Pediatric solid malignancies: Neuroblastoma and Wilms' tumor. Surgical Clinics of North America. 2006;**86**(2):469-487

[6] Kaste SC, McCarville MB. Imaging pediatric abdominal tumors. Seminars in Roentgenology. 2008;**43**(1):50-59

[7] Farmakis SG, Siegel MJ. Intrarenal neuroblastoma with pulmonary metastases mimicking a Wilms tumor. Journal of Pediatric Surgery. 2014; **49**(12):1864-1866

[8] Davenport KP, Blanco FC, Sandler AD. Pediatric malignancies. Neuroblastoma, Wilm's tumor, hepatoblastoma, rhabdomyosarcoma and sacrococcygeal teratoma. Surgical Clinics of North America. 2012;**92**(3): 745-767

[9] Rykov MY, Polyakov VG. Clinical manifestations and diagnosis of malignant neoplasms in children: What a pediatrician needs to know. The Russian Bulletin of Perinatology and Pediatrics. 2017;**62**(5):69-79. DOI: 10.21508/1027-4065-2017-62-5-69-79

[10] Metzger ML, Dome JS. Current therapy for Wilms' tumor. The Oncologist. 2005;**10**(10):815-826

[11] Fedorova DV. Differential diagnosis of neuroblastoma and Wilms' tumor. Russian Journal of Pediatric Oncology and Hematology. 2015;**4**(2):91-97. DOI: 10.17650/2311-1267-2015-2-4-91-97

[12] Agostinis P, Berg K, Cengel KA, Foster TH, Girotti AW, Gollnick SO, et al. Photodynamic therapy of cancer: An update. CA: A Cancer Journal for Clinicians. 2011;**4**(61):250-255

[13] Bacellar IOL, Tsubone TM, Pavani C, Baptista MS. Photodynamic efficiency: From molecular photochemistry to cell death. International Journal of Molecular Sciences. 2015;**9**(16):20523-20559

[14] Kessel D. Death pathways associated with photodynamic therapy. Medical Laser Application. 2006;**4**(21):219-224

[15] Mroz P, Yaroslavsky A, Kharkwal GB, Hamblin MR. Cell death pathways in photodynamic therapy of cancer. Cancers. 2011;**2**(3):2516-2539

[16] Akopov AL, Kazakov NV, Rusanov AA, Karlson A. Mechanisms of photodynamic effects in the treatment of cancer patients. Photodynamic Therapy and Photodiagnostics. 2015;**4**(2):9-16. DOI: 10.24931/2413-9432-2015-4-2-9-16

[17] Filonenko EV. Fluorescence diagnostics and photodynamic therapy—Justification of application and possibilities in oncology. Photodynamic Therapy and Photodiagnostics. 2014;**3**(1):3-7

[18] Titova VA. The role and place of PDT in multimodal treatment programs for malignant tumors. Photodynamic

Therapy and Photodiagnostics. 2012;**1**(1):3-5. DOI: 10.24931/2413-9432-2012-1-1-3-5

[19] Kumar N, Warren KB. Photodynamic therapy of dermatological conditions in pediatric population: A literature review. Photodermatology, Photoimmunology and Photomedicine. 2017;**33**(3):125-134. DOI: 10.1111/phpp

[20] Zhang B, Zhang T-H, Zheng H, Li Q, Yuan K-H, Zhi-Qi H. Therapy comparison of pulsed dye laser (PDL) and photodynamic therapy (PDT) for treatment of facial port-wine stain (PWS) birthmarks in pediatric patients. Photodiagnosis and Photodynamic Therapy. 2014;**4**(11):491-497

[21] da Silva Barbosa P, Duarte DA, Leite MF, de Sant' Anna GR. Photodynamic therapy in pediatric dentistry. Case Reports in Dentistry. 2014;**2014**(217172):5. DOI: 10.1155/2014/217172

[22] Filatova NV, Sidorenko EI, Filatov VV, Ponomarev GV, Muravyev MV. The use of photodynamic therapy with Photoditazine for the treatment of corneal neovascularization in children and adolescents. Russian Biotherapeutic Journal. 2012;**2**(11):56

[23] Rostovtsev NM, Zhukovskaya EV, Pasternak AE, Kotlyarov AN, Mustakimov BH. Morphological study of combined laser and photodynamic effect of Radachlorine on the structure of experimental Ehrlich's sarcoma. Revista Inclusions. Numero Especial. 2020. pp. 507-524

[24] Mazurin AV, Vorontsov IM. Propaedeutics of Children Diseases. Moscow: Medicine; 1985. p. 432

[25] Breslow NE. End stage renal disease in patients with Wilms tumor: Results from the National Wilms tumor Study Group and the United States Renal Data System. Journal of Urology, Nov. 2005;**174**(5):1972-1975. DOI: 10.1097/01.ju.0000176800.00994.3a

[26] Weyrich A. Survival in nephroblastoma treated according to the trial and study SIOP-9: GPOH with respect to relapse and morbidity. Annals of Oncology. 2004;**15**(5):808-820

[27] Sukhova TE. Comparative evaluation of the effectiveness of photodynamic therapy of basal cell carcinoma with intra-focal administration of Radachlorine and Photoditazine. Almanac of Clinical Medicine. 2016;**44**(1):78-87. DOI: 10.18786/2072-0505-2016-44-1-78-87

[28] Filonenko EV, Serova LG, Ivanova-Radkevich VI. Results of phase III clinical trial of the drug Radachlorine for photodynamic therapy of precancerous and primary cervical cancer. Biomedical Photonics. 2015;**4**(3):36-42. DOI: . 10.24931/2413-9432-2015-4-3-36-42

[29] Vashakmadze LA, Filonenko EV, Cheremisov VV, Khomyakov VM. Intraoperative photodynamic therapy of extra-organ retroperitoneal tumors. Photodynamic Therapy and Photodiagnostics. 2013;**2**(2):8-12

[30] Shams M, Owcharchak B, Manderscheid-Kern P, Bellnier DA, Gollnik SO. Development of photodynamic therapy regimes that control the primary tumor growth and inhibit secondary disease. Cancer Immunology, Immunotherapy. 2015;**64**:287-297

[31] Agostinis P, Berg K, Cengel KA, Foster TH, Girotti AW, et al. Photodynamic therapy of cancer: An update. CA: A cancer journal for clinicians. 2011;**61**:250-281

[32] Gollnik SO, Vaughn L, Henderson BV. Generation of effective antitumor vaccines using photodynamic

therapy. Cancer Research. 2002;**62**: 1604-1608

[33] Machinskaya EA, Ivanova-Radkevich VI. Review of the mechanisms of selective accumulation of photosensitizers of various chemical structures in tumor tissue. Photodynamic Therapy and Photodiagnostics. 2013;**2**(4):28-32

Chapter 3

Ultrasound-Guided Brachytherapy for Cervical Cancer - A Tool for Quality Improvement in Brachytherapy?

Ekkasit Tharavichitkul and Razvan M. Galalae

Abstract

Nowadays, brachytherapy is one of the major components to treat inoperable cervical cancer. Brachytherapy yields a higher dose to the target (cervix) while sparing normal tissues. Developments of brachytherapy stepped forward in the previous decade by image-guided brachytherapy (IGBT) turning brachytherapy from point-based planning to volume-based planning and IGBT improves the treatment quality for cervical cancer. Magnetic resonance imaging (MRI) or computed tomography (CT) is utilized in brachytherapy and showed promising results internationally. However, in a limited-resource area, the implementation of IGABT is difficult due to many causes (manpower, equipment, or budgets). To improve the quality in limited resources, ultrasound is introduced. The utilization of ultrasound in brachytherapy practice is to prevent uterine perforation during application. With present data, measurement by ultrasound showed the correlation to MRI measurement in uterine dimensions. With these aspects, there are many researches using ultrasound to improve the quality of treatment in brachytherapy, for example, to guide contouring on CT or to support brachytherapy planning. The use of ultrasound improves the quality of brachytherapy in comparison to conventional planning and supports the improvement in brachytherapy for cervical cancer.

Keywords: brachytherapy, cervical cancer, ultrasound

1. Introduction

Cervical cancer is one of the most common cancers among the female population with the fourth most common after breast, colorectal, and lung cancer. In 2018, there were approximately 570,000 new cases of cervical cancer with 311,000 deaths [1]. Treatment of cervical cancer is composed of surgery, radiotherapy and systemic treatment. Concurrent chemoradiation is the standard treatment for locally advanced cervical cancer (LACC) and the combination of external beam radiotherapy (EBRT) and brachytherapy (BT) maximizes the local control while minimizing the risk of toxicity. Standard EBRT should deliver a dose of 45–50.4 Gy to the whole pelvis encompassing the uterus, adnexal structures, parametria, and pelvic lymph nodes. With BT, various dose fraction schedules are used, applying a dose of 5.5–8 Gy by 3–5 fractions and the total combined dose with EBRT and BT should be in the range of 80–90 Gy [2]. From the publications of Han et al. and

Gill et al. BT is one of the major components for curative radiotherapy for LACC [3–5]. Completion of the radiation program within a suitable time is an important goal as it has a direct correlation to the outcome. The current recommendation is to finish the entire protocol of EBRT and BT within 8 weeks [2].

2. Point-based brachytherapy for cervical cancer

Brachytherapy was used to increase the curative dose to cervical cancer from the year when Todd and Meredith et al. introduced the Manchester system with radium [6, 7]. The using of point A, bladder point, and rectum point (identified in orthogonal X-rays) were reported with ICRU 38 concepts [8, 9]. The intrauterine tandem and intravaginal applicators were used in many institutes to treat cervical cancer, with acceptable results. **Figure 1** shows orthogonal X-rays for conventional planning.

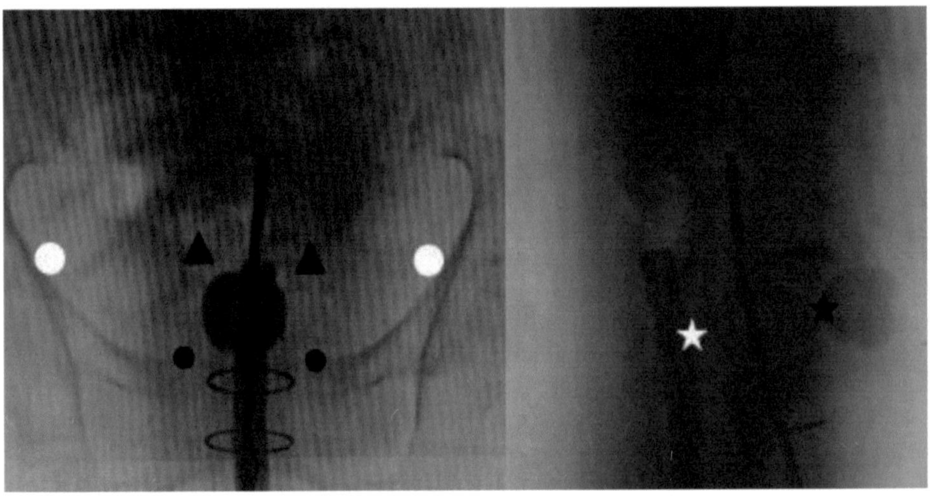

Figure 1.
Point A (black triangle), point B (white circle), ICRU bladder (black star), ICRU rectum (white star) and 5-mm vagina points (black circle) from The Division of Radiation Oncology, Department of Radiology, Faculty of Medicine, Chiang Mai University.

3. Volume-based IGBT for cervical cancer

The concepts of volume-based brachytherapy in magnetic resonance imaging (MRI) started by the publications of the Groupe European de Curietherapie and the European Society for Radiotherapy and Oncology GEC-ESTRO in 2005–2006 to propose the definitions of targets (high-risk clinical target volume; HR-CTV and intermediate-risk clinical target volume; IR-CTV) and normal tissues (Organs at risk (OARs); bladder, rectum and sigmoid) with dose constraints for evaluation [10, 11]. Moreover, the additional concepts of HR-CTV were extrapolated to CT since 2007 and developed to many international publications [12–15]. **Figure 2** shows the HR-CTV and IR-CTV according to GEC-ESTRO recommendations.

In comparison to conventional brachytherapy (point A), IGBT keeps the cumulatively curative dose to the target (HR-CTV) while sparing the cumulative dose to normal tissues [16–19]. After the first clinical results of IGBT were reported by Pötter et al. in 2007, many institutes started to develop IGBT around the world [20]. The selected publications of IGBT are shown in **Table 1** and shown promising results in local control and toxicity.

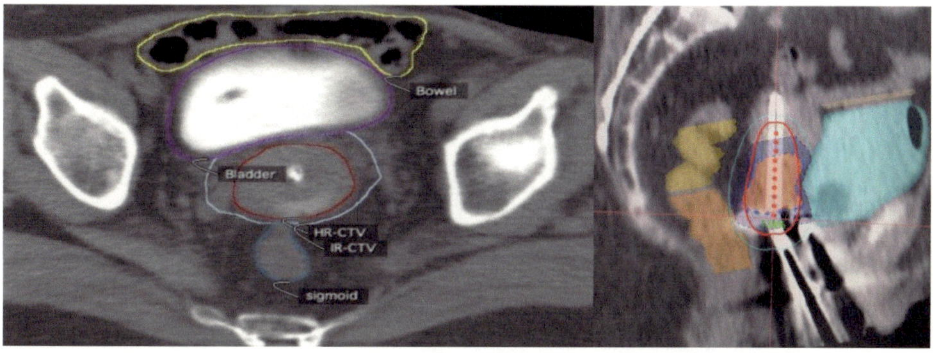

Figure 2.
HR-CTV and IR-CTV on MRI and CT related to GEC-ESTRO recommendations from the division of radiation oncology, Department of Radiology, Faculty of Medicine, Chiang Mai University.

Studies	*N*	Imaging	FU time	LC	Gr 3-4 Toxicities
Pötter et al. [21]	156	MRI	42 months	95%	11 events
Lindegaard et al. [22]	140	MRI	36 months	91%	1%(GU), 3%(GI)
Sturdza et al. [23]	731	MRI > > CT	43 months	91%	5% GU, 7% GI, 5% vagina
Tinkle et al. [24]	111	MRI with IPSA	42 months	94%	8%
Castelnau-Marchand et al. [25]	225	MRI	38.8 months	86.4%	6.6%
Mahanshetty et al. [26]	94	MRI	39 months	90.1%	3% (GU), 9%(GI)
Murakami et al. [27]	51	CT	39 months	91.7%	2% (GI)
Ohno et al. [28]	80	CT	60 months	94%	1% (GU)
Tharavichitkul et al. [29]	47	CT	26 months	97%	2.1%(GU) 2.1% (GI)
Pötter et al. [30]	1341	MRI	51 months	92%	6.8% (GU), 8.5% (GI)

BT, brachytherapy, CT, computed tomography, GI, gastrointestinal toxicity, GU, genitourinary toxicity, MRI, magnetic resonance imaging, IPSA, inverse planning simulated annealing.

Table 1.
Selected studies of IGBT.

4. Clinical results of ultrasound in brachytherapy for cervical cancer

Ultrasound in medicine was firstly developed by the military (as "sonar") and was firstly investigated in the 1940s by the method of echo-reflection to detect tumors, exudates, or abscesses [31]. Ultrasound developed very much in obstetrics and gynecology to evaluate the growing fetus and examinations in gynecological conditions [32]. Using ultrasound in clinical practice of brachytherapy divides into three aspects a) applicator guidance, b) CT-based contouring, and c) planning process. The most common use of ultrasound in brachytherapy for cervical cancer is to guide insertion of intrauterine tandem to prevent uterine perforation. Although, in this era, the incidence of uterine perforation was 3% from Segedin et al. [33]. The use of ultrasound can support accurate and safe application in brachytherapy procedures in cervical cancer. Moreover, ultrasound can help the practitioner to adjust the applicator to be a suitable position before patient transportation to the next steps. **Figure 3** shows uterine perforation by TAUS.

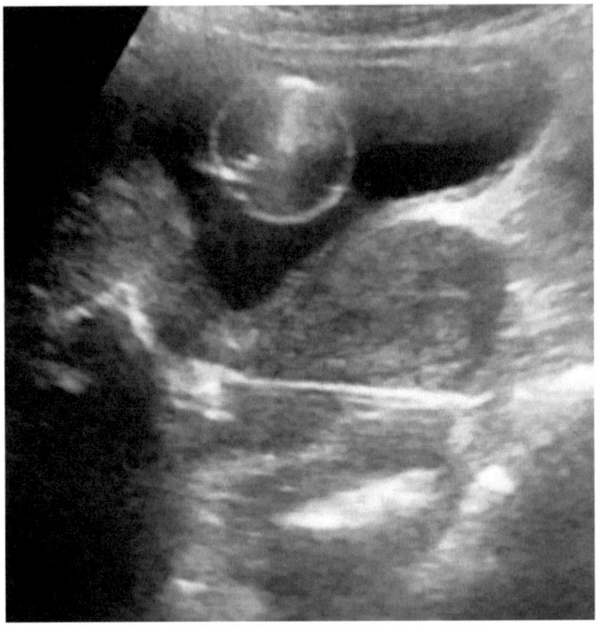

Figure 3.
Uterine perforation during insertion by TAUS from The Division of Radiation Oncology, Department of Radiology, Faculty of Medicine, Chiang Mai University.

Studies	N	Modality	Findings
Van Dyk et al. [40]	2	TAUS	TAUS is portable, nonexpensive, and simple to use and allows for accurate, conformal, re-producible, and adaptive treatments.
Van Dyk et al. [34]	71	TAUS	TAUS plan in comparison to two-dimensional MRI image was comparable for target volume ($p = 0.11$), rectal point ($p = 0.8$), and vaginal mucosa ($p = 0.19$). Local control was 90%. Late GI toxicity was less than 2%.
Mahanshetty et al. [43]	20	TAUS	TAUS correlated with MR in evaluating uterus, cervix, and central disease for IGBT.
Van Dyk et al. [35]	192	TAUS	The mean differences between TAUS and two-dimensional MRI images were less than 3 mm in the cervix. The mean differences were less than 1.5 mm at all measurement points on the posterior surface.
Narayan et al. [42]	292	TAUS	At median FU time of 41 months, 5-yr overall survival rate was 65%.
Schmid et al. [44]	19	TRUS	TRUS is better than CT as it produces systematically smaller deviations from MRI, with good to excellent image quality.
Van Dyk et al. [41]	191	TAUS	At median FU time of 5.3 years, 5-yr overall survival rate was 63%. Late toxicities were 3% for GI, 1.6% for GU, and 2% for vagina.
Mahanshetty et al. [37]	25	TRUS	CT-based delineation using MRI at diagnosis and TRUS during BT seems comparable with MRI-based approach in IGBT for cervical cancer.
Tharavichitkul et al. [45]	92	TAUS	At median FU time of 41 months, pelvic control rate was 84.8%.

BT, brachytherapy; CT, computed tomography; FU, follow up; GI, gastrointestinal; GU, genitourinary; IGBT, image-guided brachytherapy; MRI, magnetic resonance imaging; TAUS, transabdominal ultrasound; TRUS, transrectal ultrasound.

Table 2.
Selected studies showed progression of US guidance in brachytherapy.

To guide CT-based contouring is very new for using ultrasound. This comes from the pain point of CT-based contouring is an overestimation in comparison to MRI-based contouring [12]. To find the support equipment, some researchers found that the US in transabdominal (TAUS) or transrectal (TRUS) approaches showed a correlation in measurement with MRI [34–37]. Moreover, the publication from Schmid et al. showed TRUS is superior to CT as it yields systematically smaller deviations from MRI, with good to excellent image quality [38] and Mahanshetty et al. published the correlation of MRI-based contouring versus CT-based contouring supported by TRUS [37]. In recently, the latest publication from IBS-GEC ESTRO-ABS recommended TRUS to support CT-based contouring in IGBT for cervical cancer [39].

The use of TAUS in the planning process was firstly developed by Peter MacCallum Cancer Center, Melbourne, Australia [40]. This process developed from the measurement by TAUS showed a correlation to MRI [35]. In Peter MacCallum Cancer Center, the cooperation of TAUS and MRI (in first application) supported the high-end treatment in brachytherapy for cervical cancer. With this implementation, international publications were reported to support TAUS in brachytherapy [34, 35, 40, 41]. In 2014, they published a survival outcome that showed a 5-year overall survival rate of 65% [42].

The developments of US guidance for brachytherapy are concluded in **Table 2**.

5. Experiences of TAUS-guided brachytherapy in the division of radiation oncology, Department of Radiology, Faculty of Medicine, Chiang Mai University

In the Faculty of Medicine, Chiang Mai University, TAUS-guided was implemented 10 years ago to support the conventional brachytherapy during the transformation process from 2D to 3D brachytherapy since 2011. The concepts of TAUS-guided brachytherapy were adapted from Van Dyk et al. [34, 40]. From our process, we performed brachytherapy as an outpatient basis. The workflow of our procedure is shown in **Figure 4**.

After walk-in, patients were adjusted to lithotomy position and skin preparation was performed. Then, Foley's application was performed and at least 200 ml of NSS were filled into the bladder to improve the image quality of TAUS. TAUS was performed during uterine sound and intrauterine tandem applications to prevent uterine perforation. After the application finished, TAUS was performed to measure the dimension of the cervix. Eight measurements (L1-L4 and A1-A4) of cervix dimensions (from intrauterine tandem to the uterine wall) were performed (sagittal

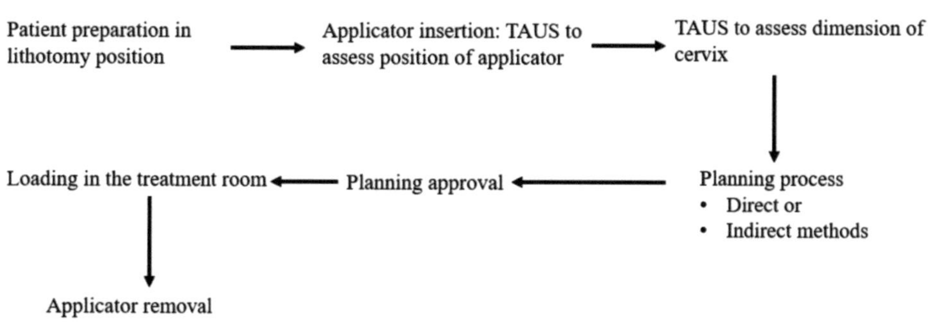

Figure 4.
Workflow of TAUS-based brachytherapy.

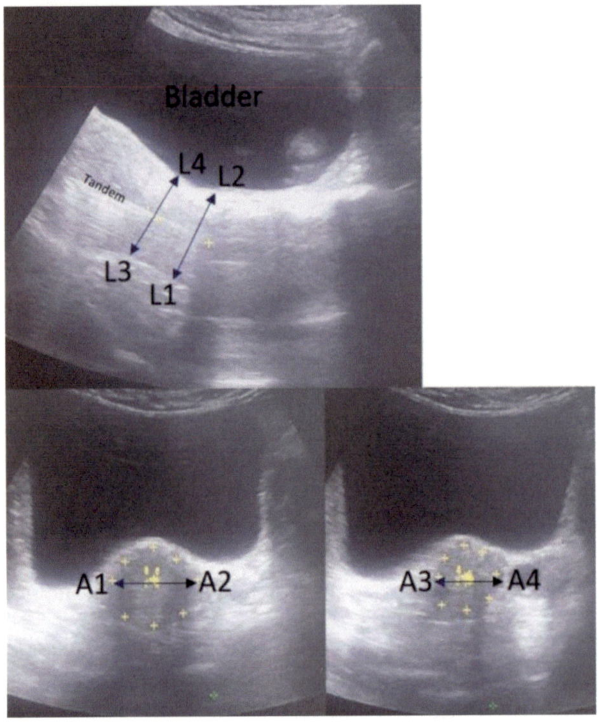

Figure 5.
Measurements in sagittal and axial views by TAUS from The Division of Radiation Oncology, Department of Radiology, Faculty of Medicine, Chiang Mai University.

and transverse approaches) at the level of the cervical OS, and 2 cm cranially to the cervical OS, adapted from previous work by Van Dyk et al. [40]. **Figure 5** shows the measurement of the cervix by TAUS.

The planning processes of TAUS-guided brachytherapy in our institute were defined as the two methods for delivering TAUS measurements into treatment planning software. When we started TAUS-guided brachytherapy in 2011, conventional brachytherapy by orthogonal X-rays was utilized by the PLATO workstation. At that time, an indirect process (to transfer the measurements from TAUS to the orthogonal X-ray) was performed. After we installed the new Oncentra workstation in 2014, a direct process (to import the DICOM images of TAUS in sagittal view to the workstation) adapted from Peter MacCallum Cancer center [34, 42] was developed to use in our patients. After applicator reconstruction by manual process or applicator library, the eight dimensions were generated to be eight cervix reference points correlated to intrauterine tandem in lateral and anteroposterior view. **Figure 6** shows the cervix reference points in the sagittal view of ultrasound sound.

After generation of eight cervix reference points, dwell weight or time was optimized to achieve a sufficiently minimal dose to the cervix reference points of at least prescribed dose (6–7 Gy per fraction). **Figure** 7 shows dose distribution by TAUS.

From our experiences, TAUS-guided brachytherapy improved the dose to the normal tissues. It reduced the cumulative overdose to the bladder (>80 Gy) and rectum (>75 Gy) in comparison to standard point A treatment and our intermediate-term results showed the 2-year local control of 88% [45]. From 2012 to 2018, more than 100 patients were treated with this technique. Nowadays, after CT was installed in our brachytherapy unit in 2019, we totally transformed to 3D (volume-based) brachytherapy. We still use TAUS to evaluate proper placement and support our CT contouring.

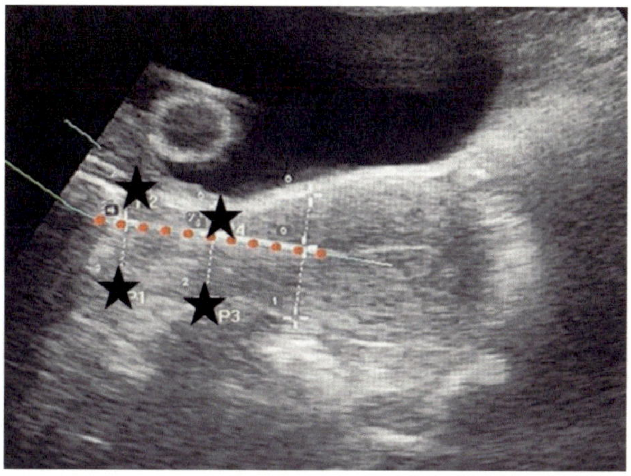

Figure 6.
TAUS images showed cervix reference points (black star) in sagittal view from The Division of Radiation Oncology, Department of Radiology, Faculty of Medicine, Chiang Mai University.

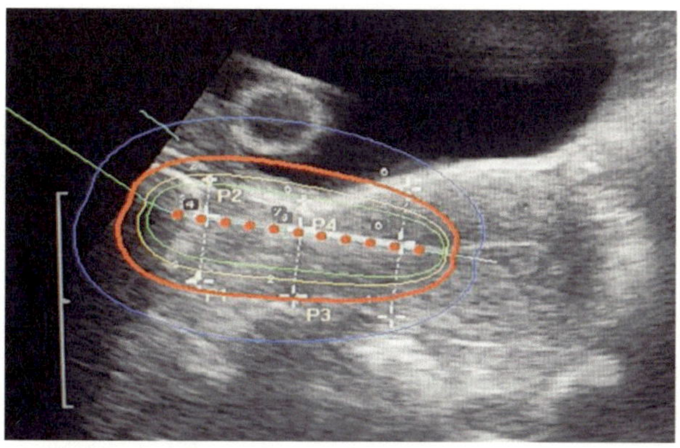

Figure 7.
Isodose distribution for TAUS-guided brachytherapy for cervical cancer (red line is 100% of prescribed dose that focus on the first 2 centimeter of uterus) from The Division of Radiation Oncology, Department of Radiology, Faculty of Medicine, Chiang Mai University.

However, TAUS still has some limitations in patients who cannot have a full bladder (cystostomy or vesicovaginal fistula), and the concept of TAUS in adaptive treatment is still on point-based planning (e.g., cervix reference points). The concept of volume-based approaches via 3D ultrasound is pending [31]. However, TAUS is inexpensive, portable, non-ionizing, and real-time equipment. TAUS supports application safely, CT contouring, and planning itself. TAUS encourages treatment quality in low-resource and high-workload centers to propose improvement in conventional brachytherapy (point A) to adaptive point-based planning (adaptive plan to cervix reference points; 2.5D). Further studies in ultrasound in CT-based contouring and planning should be performed to support the alternatives for brachytherapy in place in which MRI or CT are inaccessible.

6. Conclusion

Although trends of brachytherapy turned from point-based to volume-based plans via MRI or CT, not all cancer centers can access this equipment. To improve the quality of the point-based plan, ultrasound supports the whole process of brachytherapy, for example, applicator insertion, CT-based contouring, and planning process. TAUS-guided brachytherapy shows promising results by international publications and the cost of TAUS is cheap, and portable. Ultrasound can be applied to all levels of the cancer center to improve the quality of brachytherapy.

Acknowledgements

The author offers many thanks to all staff of the Division of Radiation Oncology, Department of Radiology, Faculty of Medicine, and Chiang Mai University for supporting all works.

Conflict of interest

The authors declare no conflict of interest.

Author details

Ekkasit Tharavichitkul[1,2*] and Razvan M. Galalae[3,4]

1 Faculty of Medicine, The Division of Radiation Oncology, Department of Radiology, Chiang Mai University, Chiang Mai, Thailand

2 Faculty of Medicine, Northern Thailand Radiation Oncology Group, Department of Radiology, Chiang Mai University, Chiang Mai, Thailand

3 MedAustron Ion Therapy Center, Wiener Neustadt, Austria

4 Faculty of Medicine, Christian-Albrechts-University, Kiel, Germany

*Address all correspondence to: ekkasit.t@cmu.ac.th

References

[1] Arbyn M, Weiderpass E, Bruni L, de Sanjosé S, Saraiya M, Ferlay J, et al. Estimates of incidence and mortality of cervical cancer in 2018: A worldwide analysis. The Lancet Global Health. 2020;**8**:e191-e203. DOI: 10.1016/S2214-109X(19)30482-6

[2] Bhatla N, Aoki D, Sharma DN, Sankaranarayanan R. Cancer of the cervix uteri. International Journal of Gynecology & Obstetrics. 2018;**143**: 22-36. DOI: 10.1002/IJGO.12611

[3] Han K, Milosevic M, Fyles A, Pintilie M, Viswanathan AN. Trends in the utilization of brachytherapy in cervical cancer in the United States. International Journal of Radiation Oncology, Biology, Physics. 2013;**87**:111-119. DOI: 10.1016/j.ijrobp.2013.05.033

[4] Gill BS, Lin JF, Krivak TC, Sukumvanich P, Laskey RA, Ross MS, et al. National cancer data base analysis of radiation therapy consolidation modality for cervical cancer: The impact of new technological advancements. International Journal of Radiation Oncology, Biology, Physics. 2014;**90**: 1083-1090. DOI: 10.1016/j.ijrobp.2014.07.017

[5] Tanderup K, Eifel PJ, Yashar CM, Pötter R, Grigsby PW. Curative radiation therapy for locally advanced cervical cancer: Brachytherapy is NOT optional. International Journal of Radiation Oncology, Biology, Physics. 2014;**88**:537-539. DOI: 10.1016/j.ijrobp.2013.11.011

[6] Tod MC, Meredith WJ. A dosage system for use in the treatment of cancer of the uterine cervix. The British Journal of Radiology. 1938;**11**:809-824. DOI: 10.1259/0007-1285-11-132-809

[7] Tod M, Meredith WJ. Treatment of cancer of the cervix uteri, a revised Manchester method. The British Journal of Radiology. 1953;**26**:252-257. DOI: 10.1259/0007-1285-26-305-252

[8] Chassagne D, Dutreix A, Almond P, Burgers JMV, Busch M, Joslin CA. 2. Definition of Terms and Concepts Currently Used in Intracavitary Therapy. Journal of the International Commission on Radiation Units and Measurements. 1985;**os-20**:4-8. DOI: 10.1093/jicru_os20.1.4

[9] Chassagne D, Dutreix A, Almond P, Burgers JMV, Busch M, Joslin CA. 3. Recommendations for Reporting Absorbed Doses and Volumes in Intracavitary Therapy. Journal of the International Commission on Radiation Units and Measurements. 1985;**os-20**: 9-14. DOI: 10.1093/jicru_os20.1.9

[10] Haie-Meder C, Pötter R, Van Limbergen E, Briot E, De Brabandere M, Dimopoulos J, et al. Recommendations from Gynaecological (GYN) GEC-ESTRO Working Group (I): Concepts and terms in 3D image based 3D treatment planning in cervix cancer brachytherapy with emphasis on MRI assessment of GTV and CTV. Radiotherapy and Oncology. 2005;**74**: 235-245. DOI: 10.1016/j.radonc.2004.12.015

[11] Pötter R, Haie-Meder C, Van Limbergen E, Barillot I, De Brabandere M, Dimopoulos J, et al. Recommendations from gynaecological (GYN) GEC ESTRO working group (II): Concepts and terms in 3D image-based treatment planning in cervix cancer brachytherapy - 3D dose volume parameters and aspects of 3D image-based anatomy, radiation physics, radiobiolo. Radiotherapy and Oncology. 2006;**78**:67-77. DOI: 10.1016/j.radonc.2005.11.014

[12] Viswanathan AN, Dimopoulos J, Kirisits C, Berger D, Pötter R. Computed tomography versus magnetic resonance imaging-based contouring in cervical

cancer brachytherapy: Results of a prospective trial and preliminary guidelines for standardized contours. International Journal of Radiation Oncology. 2007;**68**:491-498

[13] Viswanathan AN, Erickson B, Gaffney DK, Beriwal S, Bhatia SK, Lee Burnett O, et al. Comparison and consensus guidelines for delineation of clinical target volume for CT- and MR-based Brachytherapy in locally advanced cervical cancer. International Journal of Radiation Oncology. 2014;**90**:320-328

[14] Ohno T, Wakatsuki M, Toita T, Kaneyasu Y, Yoshida K, Kato S, et al. Recommendations for high-risk clinical target volume definition with computed tomography for three-dimensional image-guided brachytherapy in cervical cancer patients. Journal of Radiation Research. 2017;**58**:341-350. DOI: 10.1093/jrr/rrw109

[15] Mahantshetty U, Gudi S, Singh R, Sasidharan A, Sastri S, Gurram L, et al. Indian Brachytherapy Society Guidelines for radiotherapeutic management of cervical cancer with special emphasis on high-dose-rate brachytherapy. Journal of Contemporary Brachytherapy. 2019;**11**:293-306. DOI: 10.5114/jcb.2019.87406

[16] De Brabandere M, Mousa AG, Nulens A, Swinnen A, Van Limbergen E. Potential of dose optimisation in MRI-based PDR brachytherapy of cervix carcinoma. Radiotherapy and Oncology. 2008;**88**:217-226. DOI: 10.1016/j.radonc.2007.10.026

[17] Tharavichitkul E, Mayurasakorn S, Lorvidhaya V, Sukthomya V, Wanwilairat S, Lookaew S, et al. Preliminary results of conformal computed tomography (CT)-based intracavitary brachytherapy (ICBT) for locally advanced cervical cancer: A single Institution's experience. Journal of Radiation Research. 2011;**52**:634-640. DOI: 10.1269/jrr.10154

[18] Tharavichitkul E, Sivasomboon C, Wanwilairat S, Lorvidhaya V, Sukthomya V, Chakrabhandu S, et al. Preliminary results of MRI-guided brachytherapy in cervical carcinoma: The Chiangmai University experience. Journal of Radiation Research. 2012;**53**:313-318. DOI: 10.1269/jrr.11107

[19] Tharavichitkul E, Wanwilairat S, Chakrabandhu S, Klunklin P, Onchan W, Tippanya D, et al. Image-guided brachytherapy (IGBT) combined with whole pelvic intensity-modulated radiotherapy (WP-IMRT) for locally advanced cervical cancer: A prospective study from Chiang Mai University Hospital, Thailand. Journal of Contemporary Brachytherapy. 2013;**5**:10-16. DOI: 10.5114/jcb.2013.34338

[20] Pötter R, Dimopoulos J, Georg P, Lang S, Waldhäusl C, Wachter-Gerstner N, et al. Clinical impact of MRI assisted dose volume adaptation and dose escalation in brachytherapy of locally advanced cervix cancer. Radiotherapy and Oncology. 2007;**83**:148-155. DOI: 10.1016/j.radonc.2007.04.012

[21] Pötter R, Georg P, Dimopoulos JCA, Grimm M, Berger D, Nesvacil N, et al. Clinical outcome of protocol based image (MRI) guided adaptive brachytherapy combined with 3D conformal radiotherapy with or without chemotherapy in patients with locally advanced cervical cancer. Radiotherapy and Oncology. 2011;**100**:116-123. DOI: 10.1016/j.radonc.2011.07.012

[22] Lindegaard JC, Fokdal LU, Nielsen SK, Juul-Christensen J, Tanderup K. MRI-guided adaptive radiotherapy in locally advanced cervical cancer from a Nordic perspective. Acta Oncologica (Madr). 2013;**52**:1510-1519. DOI: 10.3109/0284186X.2013.818253

[23] Sturdza A, Pötter R, Fokdal LU, Haie-Meder C, Tan LT, Mazeron R, et al. Image guided brachytherapy in locally advanced cervical cancer: Improved pelvic control and survival in RetroEMBRACE, a multicenter cohort study. Radiotherapy and Oncology. 2016;**120**:428-433. DOI: 10.1016/j.radonc.2016.03.011

[24] Tinkle CL, Weinberg V, Chen L-M, Littell R, Cunha JAM, Sethi RA, et al. Inverse planned high-dose-rate Brachytherapy for locoregionally advanced cervical cancer: 4-year outcomes. International Journal of Radiation Oncology, Biology, Physics. 2015;**92**:1093-1100. DOI: 10.1016/j.ijrobp.2015.04.018

[25] Castelnau-Marchand P, Chargari C, Maroun P, Dumas I, Del Campo ER, Cao K, et al. Clinical outcomes of definitive chemoradiation followed by intracavitary pulsed-dose rate image-guided adaptive brachytherapy in locally advanced cervical cancer. Gynecologic Oncology. 2015;**139**:288-294. DOI: 10.1016/j.ygyno.2015.09.008

[26] Mahantshetty U, Krishnatry R, Hande V, Jamema S, Ghadi Y, Engineer R, et al. Magnetic resonance image guided adaptive Brachytherapy in locally advanced cervical cancer: An experience from a tertiary cancer center in a low and middle income countries setting. International Journal of Radiation Oncology, Biology, Physics. 2017;**99**:608-617. DOI: 10.1016/j.ijrobp.2017.06.010

[27] Murakami N, Kobayashi K, Shima S, Tsuchida K, Kashihara T, Tselis N, et al. A hybrid technique of intracavitary and interstitial brachytherapy for locally advanced cervical cancer: Initial outcomes of a single-institute experience. BMC Cancer. 2019;**19**:221. DOI: 10.1186/s12885-019-5430-x

[28] Ohno T, Noda SE, Okonogi N, Murata K, Shibuya K, Kiyohara H, et al. In-room computed tomography-based brachytherapy for uterine cervical cancer: Results of a 5-year retrospective study. Journal of Radiation Research. 2017;**58**:543-551. DOI: 10.1093/jrr/rrw121

[29] Tharavichitkul E, Chakrabandhu S, Wanwilairat S, Tippanya D, Nobnop W, Pukanhaphan N, et al. Intermediate-term results of image-guided brachytherapy and high-technology external beam radiotherapy in cervical cancer: Chiang Mai University experience. Gynecologic Oncology. 2013;**130**:81-85. DOI: 10.1016/j.ygyno.2013.04.018

[30] Pötter R, Tanderup K, Schmid MP, Jürgenliemk-Schulz I, Haie-Meder C, Fokdal LU, et al. MRI-guided adaptive brachytherapy in locally advanced cervical cancer (EMBRACE-I): A multicentre prospective cohort study. The Lancet Oncology. 2021;**22**:538-547. DOI: 10.1016/S1470-2045(20)30753-1

[31] van Dyk S, Khaw P, Lin MY, Chang D, Bernshaw D. Ultrasound-guided Brachytherapy for cervix cancer. Clinical Oncology. 2021;**33**:e403-e411. DOI: 10.1016/j.clon.2021.02.011

[32] Campbell S. A short history of sonography in obstetrics and gynaecology. Facts, Views & Vision in ObGyn. 2013;**5**:213-229

[33] Segedin B, Gugic J, Petric P. Uterine perforation - 5-year experience in 3-d image guided gynaecological brachytherapy at institute of oncology ljubljana. Radiology and Oncology. 2013;**47**:154-160. DOI: 10.2478/raon-2013-0030

[34] Van Dyk S, Narayan K, Fisher R, Bernshaw D. Conformal Brachytherapy Planning for Cervical Cancer Using Transabdominal Ultrasound. International Journal of Radiation Oncology, Biology, Physics. 2009;**75**:64-70. DOI: 10.1016/j.ijrobp.2008.10.057

[35] Van Dyk S, Kondalsamy-Chennakesavan S, Schneider M, Bernshaw D, Narayan K. Comparison of measurements of the uterus and cervix obtained by magnetic resonance and transabdominal ultrasound imaging to identify the brachytherapy target in patients with cervix cancer. International Journal of Radiation Oncology, Biology, Physics. 2014;**88**:860-865. DOI: 10.1016/j.ijrobp.2013.12.004

[36] Umesh M, Kumar DP, Chadha P, Choudary R, Kembhavi S, Thakur M, et al. Transabdominal ultrasonography-defined optimal and definitive bladder-filling protocol with time trends during pelvic radiation for cervical cancer. Technology in Cancer Research & Treatment. 2017;**16**:917-922. DOI: 10.1177/1533034617709596

[37] Mahantshetty U, Naga CHP, Khadanga CR, Gudi S, Chopra S, Gurram L, et al. A prospective comparison of computed tomography with transrectal ultrasonography assistance and magnetic resonance imaging–based target-volume definition during image guided adaptive Brachytherapy for cervical cancers. International Journal of Radiation Oncology, Biology, Physics. 2018;**102**:1448-1456. DOI: 10.1016/j.ijrobp.2018.05.080

[38] Schmid MP, Nesvacil N, Pötter R, Kronreif G, Kirisits C. Transrectal ultrasound for image-guided adaptive brachytherapy in cervix cancer – An alternative to MRI for target definition? Radiotherapy and Oncology. 2016;**120**:467-472. DOI: 10.1016/j.radonc.2016.01.021

[39] Mahantshetty U, Poetter R, Beriwal S, Grover S, Lavanya G, Rai B, et al. IBS-GEC ESTRO-ABS recommendations for CT based contouring in image guided adaptive brachytherapy for cervical cancer. Radiotherapy and Oncology. 2021;**160**:273-284. DOI: 10.1016/j.radonc.2021.05.010

[40] Van Dyk S, Bernshaw D. Ultrasound-based conformal planning for gynaecological brachytherapy. Journal of Medical Imaging and Radiation Oncology. 2008;**52**:77-84. DOI: 10.1111/j.1440-1673.2007.01917.x

[41] van Dyk S, Narayan K, Bernshaw D, Kondalsamy-Chennakesavan S, Khaw P, Lin MY, et al. Clinical outcomes from an innovative protocol using serial ultrasound imaging and a single MR image to guide brachytherapy for locally advanced cervix cancer. Brachytherapy. 2016;**15**:817-824. DOI: 10.1016/j.brachy.2016.07.008

[42] Narayan K, van Dyk S, Bernshaw D, Khaw P, Mileshkin L, Kondalsamy-Chennakesavan S. Ultrasound guided conformal brachytherapy of cervix cancer: Survival, patterns of failure, and late complications. Journal of Gynecologic Oncology. 2014;**25**:206-213. DOI: 10.3802/jgo.2014.25.3.206

[43] Mahantshetty U, Khanna N, Swamidas J, Engineer R, Thakur MH, Merchant NH, et al. Trans-abdominal ultrasound (US) and magnetic resonance imaging (MRI) correlation for conformal intracavitary brachytherapy in carcinoma of the uterine cervix. Radiotherapy and Oncology. 2012;**102**:130-134. DOI: 10.1016/j.radonc.2011.08.001

[44] Mahantshetty U, Sturdza A, Naga CHP, Berger D, Fortin I, Motisi L, et al. Vienna-II ring applicator for distal parametrial/pelvic wall disease in cervical cancer brachytherapy: An experience from two institutions: Clinical feasibility and outcome. Radiotherapy and Oncology. 2019;**141**:123-129. DOI: 10.1016/j.radonc.2019.08.004

[45] Tharavichitkul E, Chakrabandhu S, Klunklin P, Onchan W, Jia-Mahasap B, Wanwilairat S, et al. Intermediate-term results of trans-abdominal ultrasound (TAUS)-guided brachytherapy in cervical cancer. Gynecologic Oncology. 2018;**148**:468-473. DOI: 10.1016/j.ygyno.2018.01.015

Chapter 4

Treatment Practices in Optic Nerve Glioma

Rashmi Singh, Anup Kumar, Payal Raina, Rajanigandha Tudu and Praveer K.S. Munda

Abstract

Optic nerve glioma (OPG) is a rare tumor in children and adolescents. It comprises 1–5% of central nervous system tumors. It can be sporadic or associated with the neurofibromatosis 1 (*NF1*) gene. These are usually slow-growing tumors and may remain localized to the optic nerve or can have encroached upon adjoining structures like optic chiasma, opposite optic nerve, and hypothalamus. So, there may be decreased or loss of vision, proptosis, focal neurological symptoms, precocious puberty, and short stature. Due to the involvement of these critical structures, its treatment should be based on multidisciplinary consensus. The treatment modalities include surgery, RT, and chemotherapy. The aim of the treatment should be to preserve vision. However, the timing and selection of optimal treatment modalities are always a clinical dilemma. Recently, there have been promising results with newer techniques of radiotherapy and chemotherapy.

Keywords: optic nerve glioma, pediatric optic glioma, radiotherapy in optic glioma, challenges in treatment in optic glioma, optic glioma and neurofibromatosis 1

1. Introduction

Optic nerve glioma (OPG) is a rare tumor comprising 1–5% of central nervous system tumors [1]. Child and adolescent patients are most commonly affected [2]. Depending upon the tumor extent as to optic chiasma, hypothalamus, there are symptoms like vision loss, proptosis, hydrocephalous, focal neurological symptoms, precocious puberty, and short stature. Location and also, the volume of the disease are determinants of prognosis. As gliomas limited to only optic nerve (OPN) have better long-term visual outcomes than those with post-chiasmatic disease [3].

OPG has been associated with the neurofibromatosis 1 (NF1) gene in 50–60% of cases [4]. It has been observed decreased visual acuity is a more common presentation in non-NF1 patients than in NF1 positive (90% vs. 72%). However, proptosis has been found in 20–30% of cases with NF1+ and, only in 5–12% cases with non-NF1 [5].

Natural history and growth patterns have been variable for this tumor [6]. Some remain stable for years, while others demonstrate slow or rapid growth patterns.

2. Diagnosis

OPG is a radiological and clinical diagnosis. It is a type of tumor where pre-treatment tissue diagnosis is not mandatory [7]. A biopsy is limited to cases with

 IntechOpen

unusual clinical and imaging findings. Pilocytic astrocytoma is the most common histopathological variant observed, pilomyxoid astrocytoma and grade II diffuse fibrillary astrocytoma are other variants [8].

A detailed ophthalmological examination including visual clinical examination, fundoscopy, Goldmann visual field, and imaging studies (CT/MRI orbit and brain) [9], all are vital in knowing the tumor extent, response to treatment, and prognosis.

3. Treatment

The aim of the treatment should be to preserve vision. However, the timing and selection of optimal treatment modality are always a clinical dilemma [10] as it is challenging due to tumor location and treatment-related effects. Patients once diagnosed can be kept in surveillance as it remains stable for multiple years. Active intervention is to be taken once there is evidence for progression in diminition of vision or size of the tumor. Choice of the treatment to be assessed in a multidisciplinary clinic and at well-equipped centers having state of art facilities.

3.1 Surgery

Surgery can be curative when the tumor is localized to the optic nerve, [10], it can be offered as palliative treatment in advanced OPGs with no vision, and severe disfiguring proptosis. Also, as most of the time there is an involvement of optic chiasma, hypothalamus, surgery is not attempted avoid to unacceptable adverse effects.

3.2 Radiotherapy

Radiotherapy when started early this could minimize vision loss [11]. There have been reports of stabilization and also improvement in vision in the range of 13–81% post-RT [9, 12].

Long-term results of radiotherapy in a retrospective study including 89 pediatric optic-hypothalamic gliomas patients showed 10-year event-free survival (EFS) of 61.9% in NF1+ and 67.5% without NF1, whereas 10 years overall survival (OS) was 92.3%. The median dose of radiotherapy was 54 Gy/30#. However, there were reports of secondary neoplasms possibly due to RT in eight patients (four in NF1+); also, the 10-year cumulative incidence of vasculopathy was 7%. Older patients without NF1 were at low risk of toxicity [13].

So, caution should be taken while selecting patients as in children less than 6 years, where the risk of precocious puberty, growth hormone deficiency, and cerebrovascular complications has been observed in studies [14].

We have reported a case of bilateral OPG in an 18-year-old patient who was treated with intensity-modulated radiotherapy (IMRT). 54Gy/1.8 Gy/#, x 30 fractions over 6 weeks was prescribed to the planning target volume (PTV). Organs at risk (OARs) were taken care off for their tolerance. The patient had only mild irritation and watery discharge in bilateral eyes during radiotherapy with onset after 4 weeks of RT which resolved with symptomatic treatment. We observed stabilization of vision at 8 weeks follow-up [15].

In centers, where fractionated stereotactic radiotherapy (FSRT) [16] is available, the dose to the organs at risk (OARs) can be minimized by a smaller clinical target volume (CTV) margin of 1 mm and planning target volume (PTV) of 3 mm. Radiotherapy should be done by using a conformal newer technique, for example proton therapy (PRT), intensity-modulated radiotherapy (IMRT), FSRT, and Gamma knife surgery (GKS)/Cyberknife. The patient's MRI can be fused with the planning CT scan for better delineation of the tumor.

An earlier study published in 1999 by M Fuss et al. compared the dosimetric difference between PRT, 3-dimensional radiotherapy (3-D RT), and lateral photons in cases of OPG. Gross tumor volume (GTV) ranged from 3.9 cm^2 to 127 cm^2. PRT gave the advantage of covering the smallest volumes of normal tissue at all isodose levels that will extrapolate as resulting in decreased long-term toxicity. With PRT a 47–77% dose reduction to the contralateral optic nerve (OPN) was observed in comparison as to be received by 3-DRT and lateral photons. Similarly for optic chiasma and pituitary glands doses were reduced with PRT [17].

Another study involved 22 patients' majority having an extension to Chiasma/hypothalamus and five having disease limited to OPN treated with GKS. The median age of the patients was 16 years, with tumor volume 3.1 cm^3 (0.15–18.2 cm^3), prescription dose of 11.5 Gy (8–14 Gy), and mean follow-up (FU) was 43 months. Two patients were progressed, two died, the tumor shrank in 12 patients and remained stable in six patients, a controlled rate of 90% could be achieved. The authors concluded GKS to be a safe and effective treatment for OPG [18].

GKS has also shown promising results in another report where two patients of pilocytic astrocytoma of optic apparatus were treated with a dose of 11–15 Gy to 50% isodose line. Near complete response was observed in both of them at 60 months of FU [19]. Other reports using FSRT and Cyberknife in a young patient have shown a significant reduction in tumor size post-RT on FU MRI [20].

3.3 Chemotherapy

Chemotherapy has been an effective treatment in young children to preserve and stabilization of vision and delays radiotherapy [14]. It is indicated when there is a progressive disease which is evident by substantial tumor progression on MRI and or worsening of visual acuity. Although chemotherapy shrinks the tumor, up to 60% of children have tumor progression after 5 years [21].

The most common combination regimen is vincristine and carboplatin with 3–5 years progression-free survival (PFS) 77–69% respectively, although these results are from studies where the disease was extending beyond the optic nerve [22]. Other regimens with cisplatin and etoposide with 3-year PFS up to 78% have been reported [23]. In recent times monotherapy with temozolomide (TMZ) [24], vinblastine, and vinorelbine has been used for progressive or refractory disease with positive results and low toxicity. Although TMZ should be avoided in patients with NF1+.

MEK inhibitors, for example selumetinib have been reported to give 2-year PFS of 78% in a phase 2 study involving 25 patients with recurrent/progressive optic-hypothalamic gliomas. Common toxicities were grade 1–2 fatigue, asthenia, liver enzymes and creatinine phosphor kinase (CPK) elevation, diarrhea, rash, etc. [25].

OPGs are highly vascular tumors and in other tumors increased microvascular density has been associated with worse PFS. By inhibiting vascular endothelial growth factor (VEGF), neovascularization, vascular permeability, and tumor growth are inhibited with bevacizumab. In a refractory setting bevacizumab-based therapy has been reported to result in objective response and rapid improvement in visual symptoms in up to 86% of cases [26]. Adverse effects of hypertension, fatigue, bleeding have been associated with bevacizumab.

4. Conclusion

OPG is rare and difficult to treat the tumor. Improvement in vision and/or checking further progression should be the aim of selecting a treatment modality. Results with advanced techniques of radiotherapy and newer chemotherapy regimens are promising.

Acknowledgements

We acknowledge the Radiation Oncology Department staff for their support in the treatment of the patient.

Conflict of interest

None.

Financial support

None.

Author details

Rashmi Singh*, Anup Kumar, Payal Raina, Rajanigandha Tudu
and Praveer K.S. Munda
Department of Radiation Oncology, RIMS, Ranchi, India

*Address all correspondence to: rashmisingh.noor@gmail.com

References

[1] Heideman RL, Packer RJ, Albright LA, Freeman CR, Rorke LB. Tumors of the central nervous. In: Pizzo P, Poplack D, editors. Principles and Practice of Pediatric Oncology. Philadelphia (PA): Lippincott-Raven; 1997. pp. 633-697

[2] Alvord EC Jr, Lofton S. Gliomas of the optic nerve or chiasm: Outcome by patient's age, tumour site, and treatment. Journal of Neurosurgery. 1988;**68**:85-98

[3] Tow SL, Chandela S, Miller NR, Avellino AM. Long-term outcome in children with gliomas of the anterior visual pathway. Pediatric Neurology. 2003;**28**:262-270

[4] Campen CJ, Gutmann DH. Optic pathway gliomas in neurofibromatosis type 1. Journal of Child Neurology. 2018;**33**(1):73-81

[5] Jahraus CD, Tarbell NJ. Optic pathway gliomas. Pediatric Blood and Cancer. 2006;**46**(5):586-596

[6] Nicolin G, Parkin P, Mabbott D, Hargrave D, Bartels U, Tabori U, et al. Natural history and outcome of optic pathway gliomas in children. Pediatric Blood and Cancer. 2009;**53**(7):1231-1237

[7] Revere KE, Katowitz WR, Katowitz JA, et al. Childhood optic nerve glioma: Vision loss due to biopsy. Ophthalmic Plastic and Reconstructive Surgery. 2017;**33**:S107-S109

[8] Hoffman HJ, Soloniuk DS, Humphreys RP, et al. Management and outcome of low-grade astrocytomas of the midline in children: A retrospective review. Neurosurgery. 1993;**33**:964-971

[9] Tao ML, Barnes PD, Billett AL, Leong TS. Childhood optic chiasm gliomas: Radiographic response following radiotherapy and long- term clinical out- come. International Journal of Radiation Oncology, Biology, Physics. 1997;**39**:579-587

[10] Jenkin D, Angyalfi S, Becker L, Berry M. Optic glioma in children: Surveillance, resection, or irradiation? International Journal of Radiation Oncology, Biology, Physics. 1993;**25**: 215-225

[11] Flickinger JC, Torres C, Deutsch M. Management of low-grade gliomas of the optic nerve and chiasm. Cancer. 1988;**61**:635-642

[12] Grabenbauer G, Schuchardt U, Buchfelder M, Rödel CM. Radiation therapy of optico-hypothalamic gliomas (OHG)—Radiographic response, vision and late toxicity. Radiotherapy and Oncology. 2000;**54**:239-245

[13] Tsang DS, Murphy ES, Merchant TE. Radiation therapy for optic pathway and hypothalamic low-grade gliomas in children. International Journal of Radiation Oncology, Biology, Physics. 2017;**99**(3):642-651

[14] Janss AJ, Grundy R, Cnaan A, Savino PJ. Optic pathway an hypo-thalamic/chiasmatic glioma in children younger than age 5 years with a 6-year follow-up. Cancer. 1995;**75**:1051-1059

[15] Singh R, Kumar A, Tudu R, Raina P, Munda P. IMRT in a rare case of bilateral optic nerve glioma. Journal of Radiotherapy in Practice. 2021;**20**(1): 120-122

[16] Combs S, Schulz D, Moschos D, Thilmamm C. Fractionated stereotactic radiotherapy of optic pathway gliomas: Tolerance and long-term outcome. International Journal of Radiation Oncology, Biology, Physics. 2005;**62**: 814-819

[17] Fuss M, Hug EB, Schaefer RA, Nevinny-Stickel M, Miller DW, Slater JM, et al. Proton radiation therapy (PRT) for pediatric optic pathway gliomas: Comparison with 3D planned

conventional photons and a standard photon technique. International Journal of Radiation Oncology, Biology, Physics. 1999;**45**(5):1117-1126

[18] El-Shehaby AM, Reda WA, Abdel Karim KM, Emad Eldin RM, Nabeel AM. Single-session Gamma Knife radiosurgery for optic pathway/ hypothalamic gliomas. Journal of Neurosurgery. 2016;**125**(Suppl 1):50-57

[19] Liang CL, Lu K, Liliang PC, Chen HJ. Gamma Knife surgery for optic glioma. Report of 2 cases. Journal of Neurosurgery. 2010;**113**:44-47

[20] Uslu N, Karakaya E, Dizman A, Yegen D, Guney Y. Optic nerve glioma treatment with fractionated stereotactic radiotherapy. Journal of Neurosurgery: Pediatrics. 2013;**11**(5):596-599

[21] Kelly JP, Leary S, Khanna P, Weiss AH. Longitudinal measures of visual function, tumor volume, and prediction of visual outcomes after treatment of optic pathway gliomas. Ophthalmology. 2012;**119**(6):1231-1237

[22] Packer RJ, Ater J, Allen J, et al. Carboplatin and vincristine chemotherapy for children with newly diagnosed progressive low-grade gliomas. Journal of Neurosurgery. 1997;**86**:747-754

[23] Massimino M, Spreafico F, Cefalo G, et al. High response rate to cisplatin/ etoposide regimen in childhood low-grade glioma. Journal of Clinical Oncology. 2002;**20**:4209-4216

[24] Gururangan S, Fisher MJ, Allen JC, et al. Temozolomide in children with progressive low-grade glioma. Neuro-Oncology. 2007;**9**:161-168

[25] Fangusaro J, Onar-Thomas A, Poussaint TY, Wu S, et al. A phase 2 trial of selumetinib in children with recurrent optic pathway and hypothalamic low-grade glioma without NF1: A pediatric brain tumor consortium study. Neuro-Oncology. 2021;**23**(10):1777-1788

[26] Hwang EI, Jakacki RI, Fisher MJ, et al. Long-term efficacy and toxicity of bevacizumab-based therapy in children with recurrent low-grade gliomas. Pediatric Blood and Cancer. 2013;**60**: 776-782

Chapter 5

The Remodeling in Cancer Radiotherapy

Ion Christian Chiricuta

Abstract

Remodeling is a new concept used to describe the effects of cancer cells properties to modify the extracellular microenvironment (ECM) to favor the proliferation, invasiveness, migration, and metastatic potential of the tumor. All these characteristics are determined by both the direct and indirect interactions of the cancer cells, with components of their microenvironment. The remodeling concept described in this chapter considers the changes produced by the local treatment alone, or in combination with systemic treatments on local advanced primary tumors or bone metastases (vertebral body or pelvic bones). The cases presented considered locally advanced cancer that disturbed the local anatomy at different levels as chest wall, the skin of the face, eye orbit, and vertebral or pelvic bones. Changes in the extracellular microenvironment, after the applied treatment, normalized all or only in special parts of the extracellular matrix, with a remodeling organ-specific process to the treated tumor bed. In some of these cases was reached a restitutio till to the most important component, the basal membrane. The four phases of the healing process of lesions produced by radiotherapy (the hemostasis, inflammatory, proliferative, and remodeling phase) and the possible changes at the level of ECM were here analyzed.

Keywords: remodeling, radiotherapy, extracellular microenvironment, locally advanced cancer, restitutio ad integrum, healing process

1. Introduction

There has been a massive shift in our approach to understand the biology of solid tumors in the last decades. While research centered for a long time nearly exclusively on the individual tumor cells, the process leading to their transformation, or conveying their malignancy, and the tumor as a complex organ, meanwhile the term tumor microenvironment (TME) is used, to describe the entirety of the tumor components that are not malignant by themselves. Thus, the TME consists of the tumor vasculature, connective tissue, infiltrating immune cells, and the extracellular matrix (ECM). Increasingly, all these individual components of the TME became the focus of new research communities within the fast-growing cancer field. The ECM is probably the component of the TME that initially received the least attention, but this also changed considerably over the last decade. The numerous articles have, bit by bit, complemented our understanding of the tumor ECM and its role in malignancy and response to therapy [1].

Cancer represents a dysregulation of the body's normal, controlled cellular programs. Malignant cells are able to confer enhanced proliferation, resistance to apoptosis, or motility that allows tumors to metastasize (colonize) the distant organs, which is the most lethal aspect of cancer. Tumor cells also require the collaboration of the tumor microenvironment (TME) for growth and progression [2].

Tumor hypoxia or increased inflammation in the TME modifies tumor ECM components and increases collagen deposition, ECM density, and stiffness. In addition, it is known that adhesion to the dense ECM modifies the radiation sensitivity of cancer cells.

Radiotherapy is considered as one of the potentially curative modalities for cancer. The tumor ECM might play a pivotal role in resistance and recurrences to radiotherapy in different cancers.

2. Remodeling as part of cancer development

Recent concepts of ECM remodeling shaping tissues for tumor cells to invade and metastasize during cancer development are discussed in the literature. Increasing understanding of these processes opens up the possibilities of therapeutic approaches to target the aberrant ECM and/or the underlying pathologic mechanisms of its remodeling and prevent malignancy. Changing single elements can turn over the delicate balance of ECM remodeling events.

It is not surprising that cancer cells modify all four ECM remodeling mechanisms, creating a cancer-supporting matrix that actively contributes to the pathology of the tumor.

The tumor microenvironment regulates cancer initiation, progression, and response to therapy. The immature tumor vasculature may impede drugs from reaching tumor cells at a lethal concentration. Potiron et al. [3] have shown that RT-induced vascular remodeling translates into improved tissue distribution and efficacy of chemotherapy.

Radiotherapy (RT) induces vascular remodeling, accompanied by decreased hypoxia and/or increased perfusion. In a low dose regime (2 Gy/fraction) it is a common effect. Intra-tumoral doxorubicin distribution was improved.

These data demonstrate that RT favors the efficacy of chemotherapy by improving tissue distribution and could be an alternative chemo sensitization strategy.

Even in the era of targeted therapies, the limited distribution of drugs remains a challenge. This is part of the abnormal tumor vasculature, which has developed as a function of anarchic tumor expansion. The resulting network is tortuous, overbranched, variable in diameter, and abnormally permeable [3]. The consequence is reduced blood flow. Additional tumor cell density creates a compressive environment that blunts the endothelial lumen and limits the extravasation of molecules because of high interstitial pressure. The abnormal vasculature generates hypoxia and acidosis, leading to metabolism switch and the emergence of therapeutic resistance. Moreover, destructing angiogenesis or altering vascular maturation could favor metastasis.

External radiotherapy is today a standard treatment for about half of cancer patients, either alone or in combination with surgery and/or chemotherapy, given in a fractionated regimen of about 2 Gy/day, over a course of several weeks, to achieve a total dose of 32–80 Gy, depending on tumor type and location. Endothelial deaths after irradiation might be trigger only above 5–10 Gy.

Ultimately, RT leads to the destruction of target tissues. However, this process is gradual and allows time for complex biological phenomena to occur. Potiron et al. [3] have shown in a xenograft prostate model that RT induces perivascular coverage of tumor micro-vessels.

Pericytes belong to a versatile cell population, whose function and origin are still under debate. Their interaction with endothelial cells is dynamic during vascular development and maturation. The lack of pericytes impairs vascular function and favors metastasis. Whether pericytes contribute to upregulating perfusion in a radiotherapy context is not completely elucidated. The function of pericytes in regulating blood flow is currently questioned [3].

3. Target volume definition, clinical target volume, and radiotherapy

The treatment of locally advanced cancers patients is a subject of debate in the last decades. A complex treatment including surgery, chemotherapy, hormone therapy, and radiotherapy is a standard today. New concepts had to be developed since the progress in diagnostic methods, tumor characterization, and progress in treatment delivery (more aggressive surgery and radiotherapy) made possible new approaches for locally advanced cancers.

In recent decades, tumor imaging by the introduction of computer tomography (CT), magnetic resonance imaging (NMR), and of positron emission tomography (PET/CT) made possible real progress in radiotherapy. From the 2D radiotherapy standard routine, for example, in breast cancer radiotherapy, a transition to 3D radiotherapy was possible. The high frequency of acute and late side effects to the normal structures around the real target volume (the breast tissue, chest wall, and lymphatic areas as axilla, internal mammary chain, and supraclavicular lymph nodes) made necessary new developments. The most important step forward was realized by the introduction of the concept of the anatomical defined clinical target volume (CTV) which included the microscopical disease and the gross tumor volume regarding the macroscopic visible tumor (GTV). The normal tissues around the above-defined target volumes were the loco-regional lymphatics (axillary nodes, internal mammary chain node, and the supraclavicular lymphatics), the brachial plexus, the lung tissue, the myocardium, and the ribs are so, well visualized. The concept of target volumes and real advanced conformal radiotherapy to apply the necessary curative dose to the CTV and GTV and to reduce the dose delivered to the organs of risk was developed and routinely applied, in the late eighties, by the team conducted by professor W. Bohndorf at the University of Würzburg, Germany. The initial concept of target volume definition was published by Richter and Bohndorf [4]. The development of conformal irradiation techniques to cover the CTV and GTV and to reduce the applied dose to the organs at risk was realized by the department of medical physics conducted by professor Richter (**Figure 1**) [6].

Reducing the irradiated volume by irradiation of a well-defined GTV (gross tumor volume) and CTV (clinical target volume) made it possible for the application of larger total dose of irradiation and a reduction of the acute and late side effects. These irradiated volumes included the tumor microenvironment (TME) which contains the tumor cells and the remodeled tissue now defined as the extracellular microenvironment (ECM).

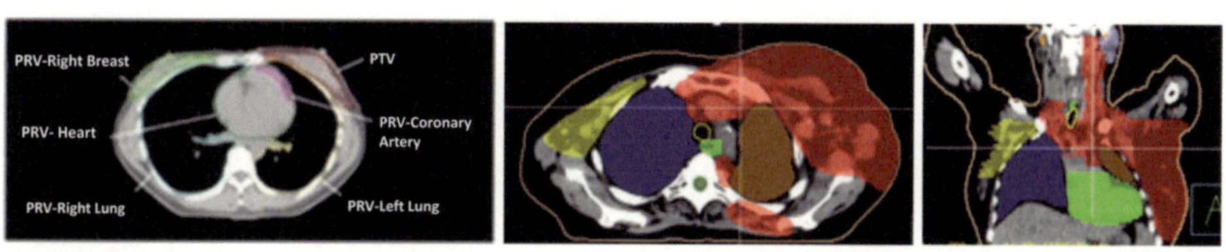

Figure 1.
PTV (planning target volumes) (left side), [5] and CTV and GTV and the organs at risk (middle and right side) for advanced breast cancer radiotherapy [6].

4. Extracellular matrix in the tumor microenvironment and its impact on cancer therapy

Solid tumors are complex organ-like structures, that consist not only of tumor cells but also of the vasculature, extracellular matrix (ECM), stromal, and immune cells. Often, this tumor microenvironment (TME) comprises the larger part of the overall tumor mass. Like the other components of the TME, the ECM in solid tumors differ significantly from that of normal organs. Intra-tumoral signaling, transport mechanisms, metabolisms, oxygenation, and immunogenicity are strongly affected if not controlled by the ECM. Exerting this regulatory control, the ECM does not only influence the malignancy and growth of the tumor but also its response toward therapy. Understanding of particularities of the ECM in the solid tumor is required to develop approaches to interfere with its negative effect.

In this chapter, we will also highlight the current understanding of the physical, cellular, and molecular mechanisms by which the pathological tumor ECM affects the efficiency of radiotherapy [1].

The effect of ionizing radiation on cells is also strongly dependent on their oxygenation status. Hypoxia significantly impairs the effectiveness of radiotherapy.

5. Remodeling, cellular aspects at the level of the extracellular matrix

The influence of ionizing radiation at the tumor tissue and cell level and the processes of reducing the side effects of radiation are schematically represented in **Figure 2**.

At the top of the image are represented the four phases of the healing process of lesions produced by surgery or radiotherapy namely the phase of hemostasis, inflammatory phase, proliferative phase, and the remodeling phase.

At the bottom of the image are shown schematically the biological processes as a result of the action of radiation on the tumor DNA and due to double-stranded lesions that are irreversible, which finally facilitates the destruction of tumor cells by initiating the process of cell death called apoptosis. This explains how local tumor control is possible. Optimizing this process of tumor destruction and restoring the structures of the peritumoral tissue makes possible the remodeling process in which the healing process is present [6].

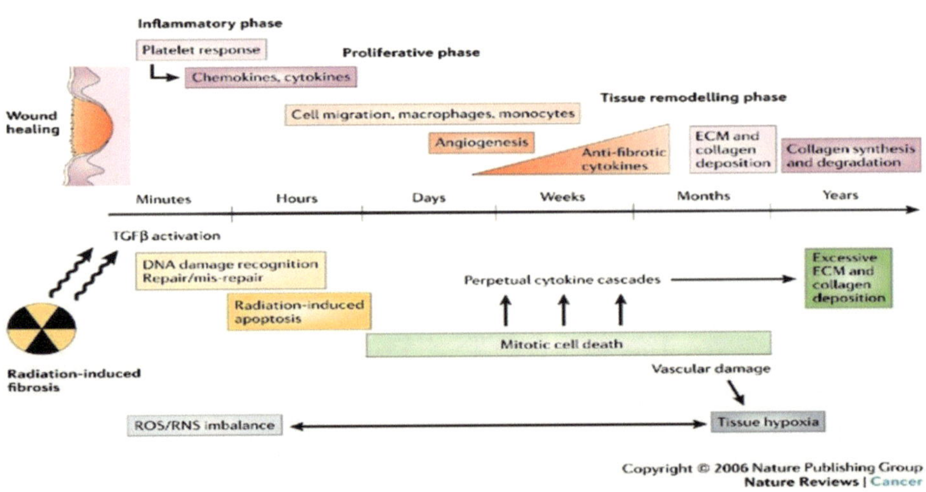

Figure 2.
Schematic representation of radiation action at the tumor cell level (at the bottom) and of the remodeling and scarring process (at the top of the figure) [7].

The role of the extracellular matrix and cellular regulators in the plasticity of tumor cells are schematically rendered in **Figure 3**. The destruction of the tumor following irradiation makes it possible to restore the basal membrane and sometimes even remodeling with restitutio ad integrum in the tumor bed is possible.

Tissue restoration ad integrum after the destruction of malignant tumor and restoration of the basal membrane is shown below [6].

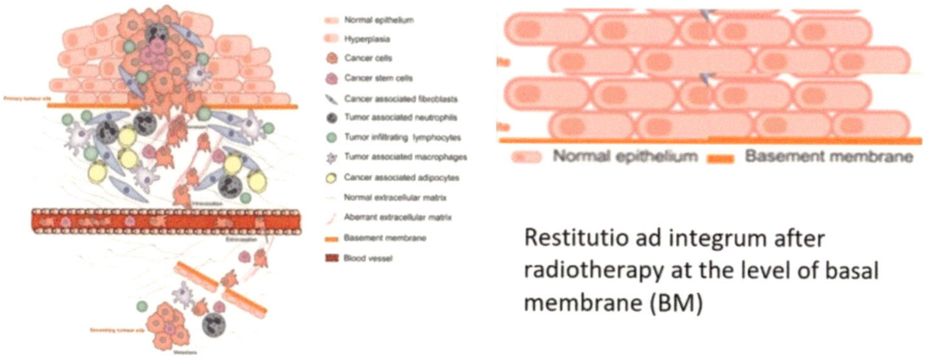

Figure 3.
Schematic representation of pathophysiological processes that demonstrate the cellular plasticity of tumor cells in the invasion process with tumor progression and metastasis (on the left side) [8] and restoration of the basal membrane and epithelium after tumor destruction by irradiation (on the right side).

6. Remodeling of normal tissue to TME

In the next three pictures, we visualize the remodeling process from "normal" ECM of the normal state of the rectum to the appearance of the tumor microenvironment (TME), with two well-defined parts: the proliferative well-vascularized peripheral one and a central necrotic part (in the middle). Six weeks after neoadjuvant radio-chemotherapy, a partial remission with a complete disappearance of the well-vascularized macroscopic part of the tumor was reached (right) and a remnant scar at the site of the necrotic part of the treated primary rectal cancer was noted.

The representation of the complex process from a normal rectal mucosa state (left picture) to the state in which rectal cancer with its central necrotic part and the peripheral well-vascularized part (in the middle), under neoadjuvant radio-chemotherapy was reduced to scar tissue (right picture) is shown in **Figure 4**. This is the visualized tumor response after 56 Gy was applied in 28 fractions on the macroscopic visible tumor (in the middle). The histologic examination of the scar revealed only remnant tumor cells in the lymphatics (LVI). One year later, the patient developed multiple brain metastases.

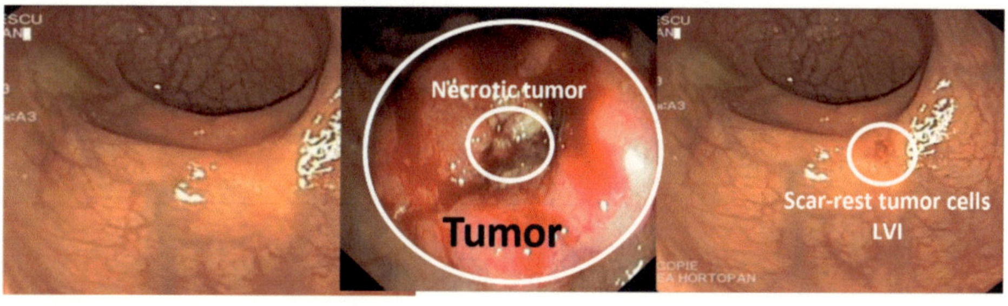

Figure 4.
Normal rectal mucosa before tumor appearance (left), with macroscopic tumor (middle) and 6 weeks after radio-chemotherapy (right) and before surgery.

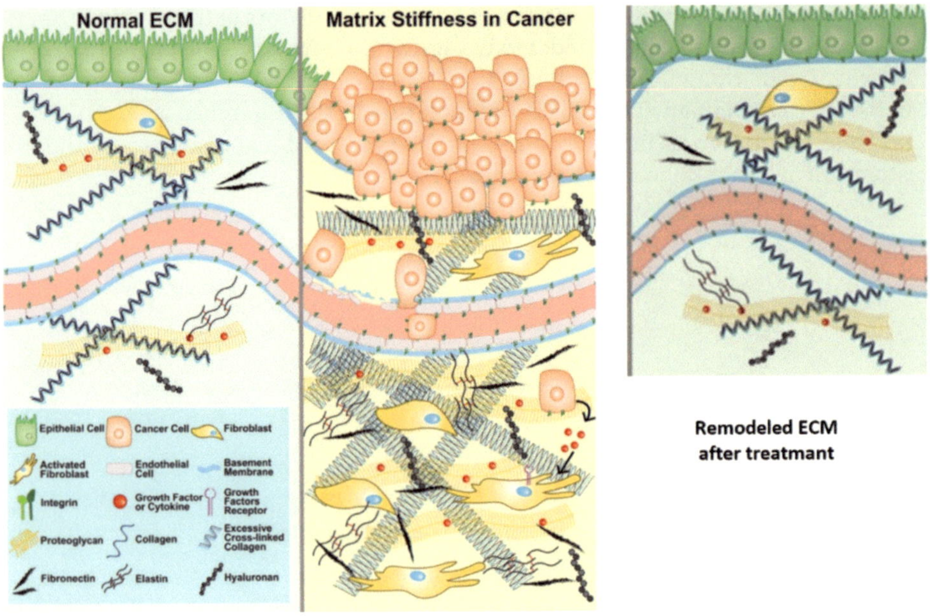

Figure 5.
Schematic representation of the ECM in normal tissue (left), TME in tumor tissue (middle), and ECM modified after radiation therapy (right) [1].

Above is a schematic representation of the ECM at the level of the normal rectum (left side), of the tumor microenvironment (TME) of the rectal tumor (in the middle), and the "remodeled" TME with the complete destruction of the tumor now "remodeled ECM" and a recovered basal membrane (right side) (**Figure 5**).

The "Remodeled" ECM after treatment became more abundant, denser, stiffer, with more fibroblasts and collagen.

7. Wound healing and tissue repair process

Besides the tumor destruction by radiotherapy which includes the remodeling process to normalize the ECM, in which the tumor cells were killed, an additional process defined as wound healing, that includes the process of restauration of the processes produced by the irradiation of the normal tissues around the tumor, or in the tumor bed, described as acute and late side effects is present.

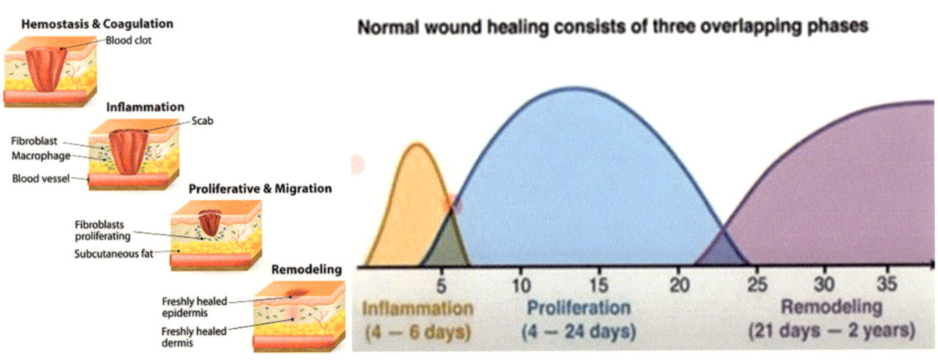

Figure 6.
Left side: Stages of the process of healing after surgery and radiotherapy with their overlapping (on the time scale): Inflammatory phase, proliferation, and tissue remodeling with collagen accumulation in the terminal phase [9]. Right side: Overlapping of wound healing [10].

The complexity of the "healing" after surgery and the tissue repair process after radiotherapy, with the representation of the 4 phases of healing that are partially overlapping, is shown in the figure (**Figure 6**).

8. "Remodeling" at the vascular level of malignant tumors

The local tumor progression is also facilitated by the production of a new vascularization with "neogenesis vessels" as shown in **Figure 7**. The neoformation vessels have an increased permeability, that facilitates the process of remote metastasis. At the tumor level occur several processes such as angiogenesis, lymph angiogenesis, vascular permeability, and all the consequences of these processes (tumor hypoxia, vascular fragility, aggressiveness) [6].

The action of radiotherapy at the level of tumor vascularization allows a normalization, that is, a vascular "remodeling" with all the advantages resulting from

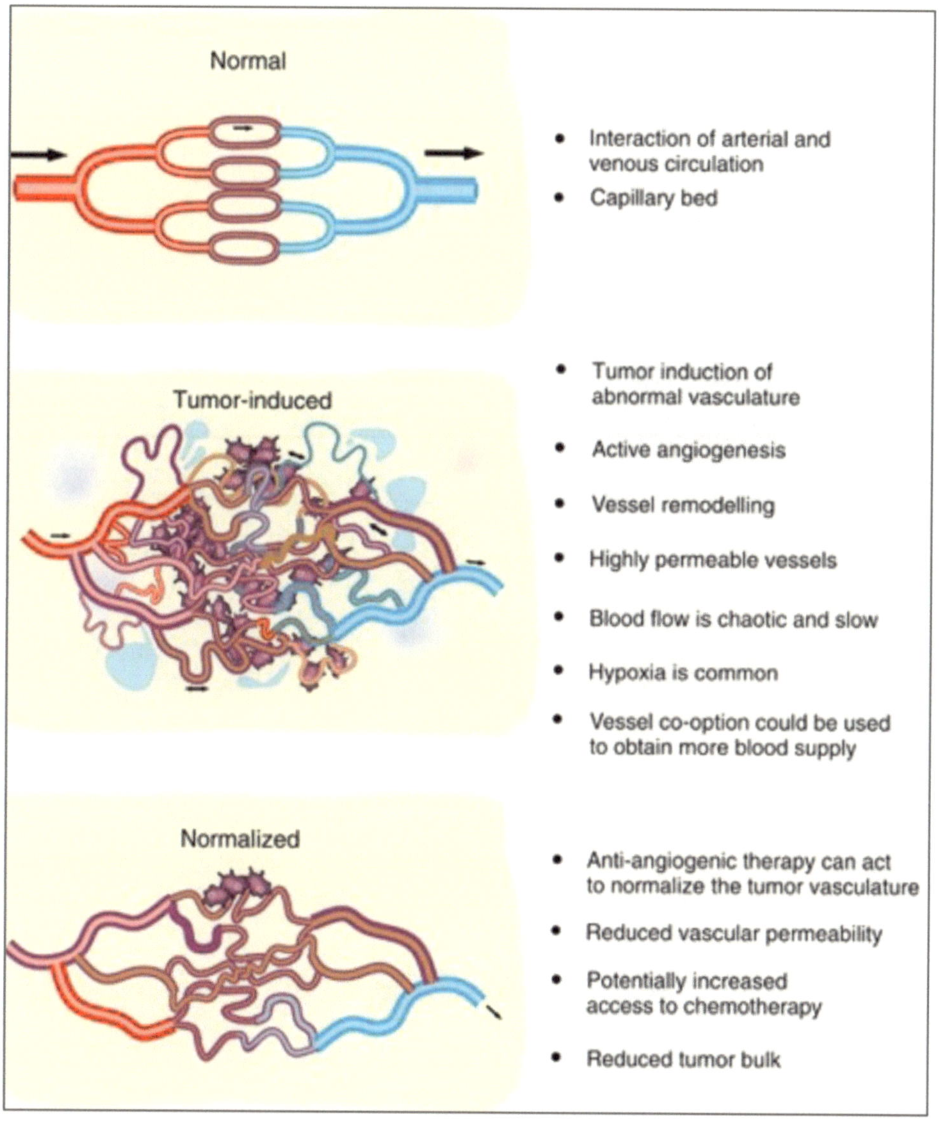

Figure 7.
Processes induced at the tumor vascular level and the possible vascular "normalization" through therapy (chemotherapy and radiotherapy) [2].

it (better oxygenation of tissues, more efficient action of cytostatics and radiation, reduction of hemorrhages).

9. Clinical aspects of remodeling

9.1 Remodeling of a skin tumor

We present here the clinical evolution of a basal cell carcinoma (basalioma) located on the face of a 100-year-old patient (**Figure 8**).

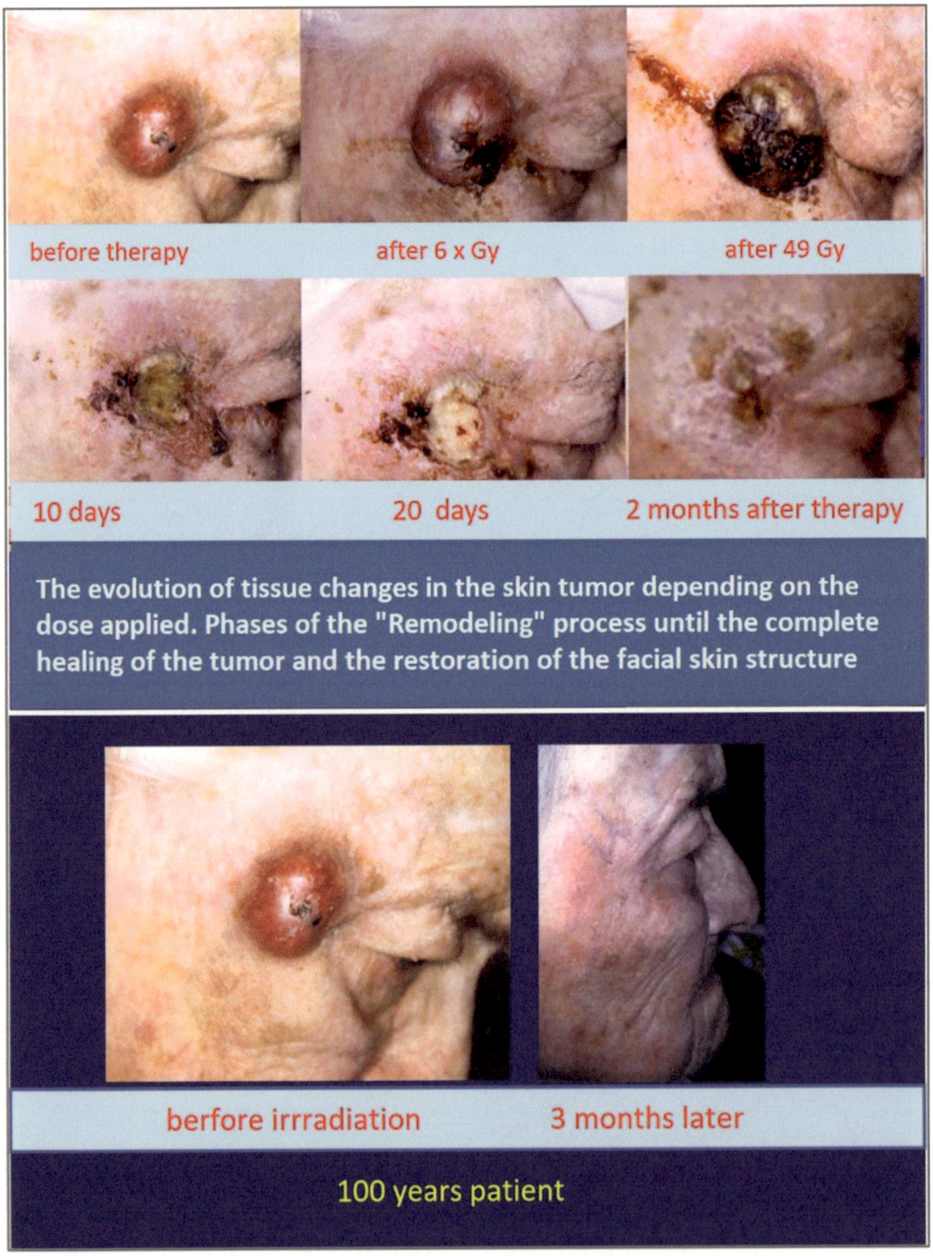

Figure 8.
The evolution of the remodeling of a basal cell carcinoma at the level of the right temple. Tumor before and during the application of local electron radiotherapy (flap applied to the irradiated area). After applying the first seven fractions of 2 Gy, the next 6 days were applied two daily fractions of 3 Gy (6 hours apart). The last 10 fractions of 2 Gy were applied until the total dose of 70 Gy was reached.

This case demonstrates the ability of "remodeling" at the level of this skin tumor and of the healthy peritumoral tissue, when the primary tumor is irradiated with a high total dose and fractionation that allows tumor control and does not produce side effects on these structures at high risk of the applied dose. In this case, the healing action was initiated and completed by the activity of macrophages and the stimulation of fibroblasts present at this level with a role in limiting side effects.

The action of fibroblasts contributed to the remodeling process with a favorable final result, in which not the slightest signs of scarring can be seen. Thus, it was possible to "remodel" at this level all the structures initially involved and disturbed through the tumor process. The skin, including the basal membrane, was completely restored, without the formation of a scar, acute skin side effects have been reduced.

9.2 Remodeling of an orbital tumor

The treatment of patients with advanced local orbital and facial cancer has been a much-debated topic in recent decades. At the end of the last decade, the complex treatment has included radical surgeries such as enucleation, reconstructive plastic surgery, chemotherapy, and radiation therapy. All these interventions were accompanied by accentuated side effects. New concepts could be developed due to advances in the diagnostic methods, tumor characterization, and the progress in the application of treatment (conservative surgery or high-dose radiotherapy) for cancer located in the orbit and the soft parts of the face.

We are going to present here the clinical evolution of an orbital advanced cancer and infiltration of the facial skin, in a 90-year-old patient, who presented in our department. This patient was treated with IMRT radiotherapy (intensity-modulated radiotherapy) with TOMOTHERAPY at the POLISANO Radiotherapy Center, Sibiu. Histopathological and immunohistochemical examination classified the lymphoma as a B-cells non-Hodgkin's lymphoma (NHL). The patient had two locations, one on the right orbita and the other suborbital and paranasal on the left side. Both locations were irradiated at the same time. A complete clinical remission was obtained for both locations.

The frequency of orbital tumors is low, representing only 0.1% in general and only 20% of all orbital diseases. The most common type of orbital tumor is non-Hodgkin's lymphoma. It generally manifests at the level of the ocular appendages, in 45–75% of cases being the extranodal lymphoma of the marginal area. Follicular lymphoma occurs in 15–30% of cases and diffuse B-cell lymphoma occurs in only 10% of cases. From a topographic point of view in 30–80% of cases, the conjunctiva is affected, in 10–50% the retrobulbar tissue, and in 10–55% the lacrimal gland. Radiotherapy is the method of choice in the treatment of orbital lymphomas. Multiple studies have reported satisfactory results by applying total doses between 24 and 46 Gy in standard fractionation with 1.8–2.0 Gy per fraction. The average total dose applied is 32 Gy.

The anatomy of the orbit and the extreme radio sensitivity of the various components of the orbit are a challenge for radiotherapy and radiotherapist. The orbital tumors occupy the space between the eyeball and the bony wall of the orbit. These include tumors of the eye that invade the orbit as well as ancillary structures such as sinuses, orbital bones, and the central nervous system.

9.2.1 Radiotherapy of an orbital tumor

The case of the 90-year-old patient demonstrates the capacity of "remodeling" that exists in healthy peritumoral tissues when the primary tumor is irradiated with a high total dose and fractionation that allows tumor control and does not produce side effects in organs and structures at high risk at the applied dose. In this case, the healing action was initiated and completed by the activity of macrophages and the stimulation of fibroblasts present at this level with a role in limiting side effects. The action of fibroblasts contributed to the remodeling process with a favorable final result, in which not the slightest signs of scarring are seen. So, it was possible to "remodel" at this level all the structures initially involved in the tumor process: the patient's eyeball with the soft parts of the orbit and the facial skin. The skin is completely restored without the formation of a scar. Acute skin side effects have been reduced.

In the healing process, the role of macrophages is to remove damaged tumor cells by double-stranded damage to tumor DNA. In this case, the process of fibrosis at the level of the tumor bed was not noticed. The target volume had two components, namely the macroscopic tumor evaluated by imaging using a CT examination with and without a contrast agent and an MRI examination, also with and without a contrast agent. The irradiation plan was performed and subsequently applied at a TOMOTHERAPY machine (Polisano Center in Sibiu) developed under the instructions of Dr. Adrian Moga.

There is a wide spectrum of radiation tolerance between the various components of the orbital region. While the lens and the lacrimal gland are the most sensitive and their functionality is profoundly affected by doses above 10 Gy in standard fractionation, other structures such as the optic nerve tolerate doses up to 40–46 Gy.

The initiation of the radiological treatment was performed by performing a CT examination with the necessary means of contention. The irradiation plan with

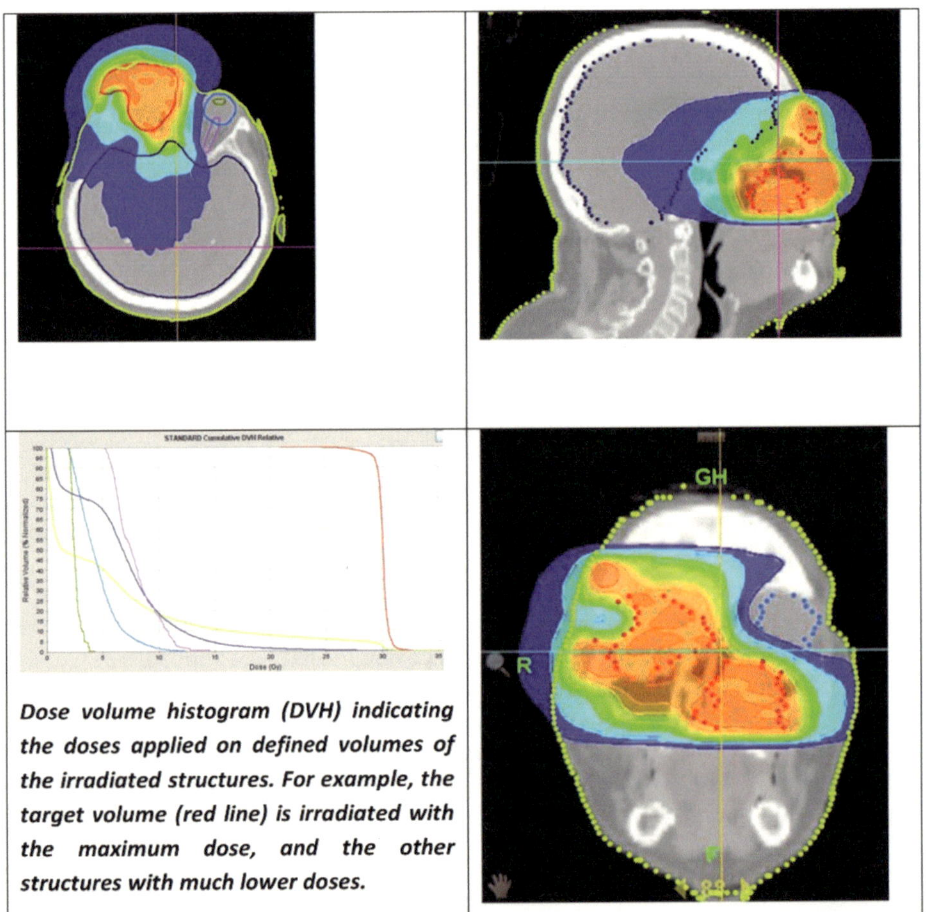

Figure 9.
Delineation of the macroscopic tumor masses by GTV (gross tumor volume) corresponding to the two tumor manifestations (right orbit and left suborbital and paranasal lesion). Irradiation plan with isodose distribution and volume dose histogram (DVH). The macroscopic tumor (GTV) obtains the maximum dose over the entire volume while the OR (organs at high risk of irradiation) such as the right and left eyeballs are underdosed, thus being protected to the maximum.

the information on the applied doses and at the level of the so-called radiosensitive structures DVH (dose-volume histogram) are reproduced in **Figure 9**.

The response to radiotherapy of the 90-year-old patient with an orbital tumor, non-Hodgkin's lymphoma, manifested in the soft parts of the face and the right orbit, with the initial clinical situation until the complete response after radiotherapy is shown in **Figure 10**.

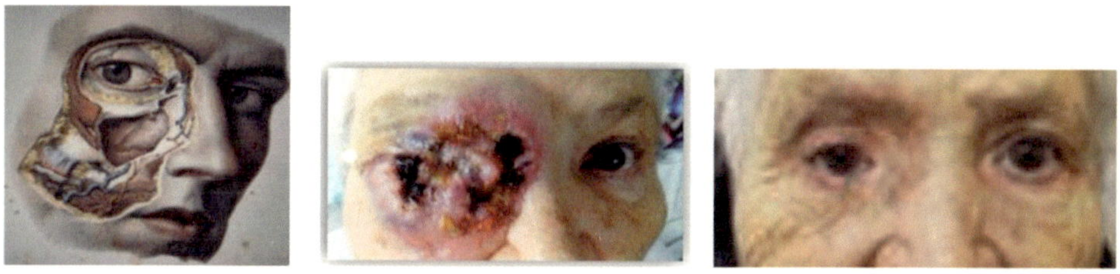

Figure 10.
Left: Anatomical details at the level of the orbit and of the cheek. Right: Orbital tumor and invasion of the skin of the face (peritumoral infiltrative process and huge area of necrosis) before starting the radiation and after completion of radiation therapy with "Remodeling" ad integrum (preserved own eyeball).

9.3 Remodeling of a locally advanced breast cancer

We present here the clinical situation of a local advanced breast cancer in women aged 82 who presented in our department and was treated by a conformal 10 fields of radiotherapy (**Figure 11**).

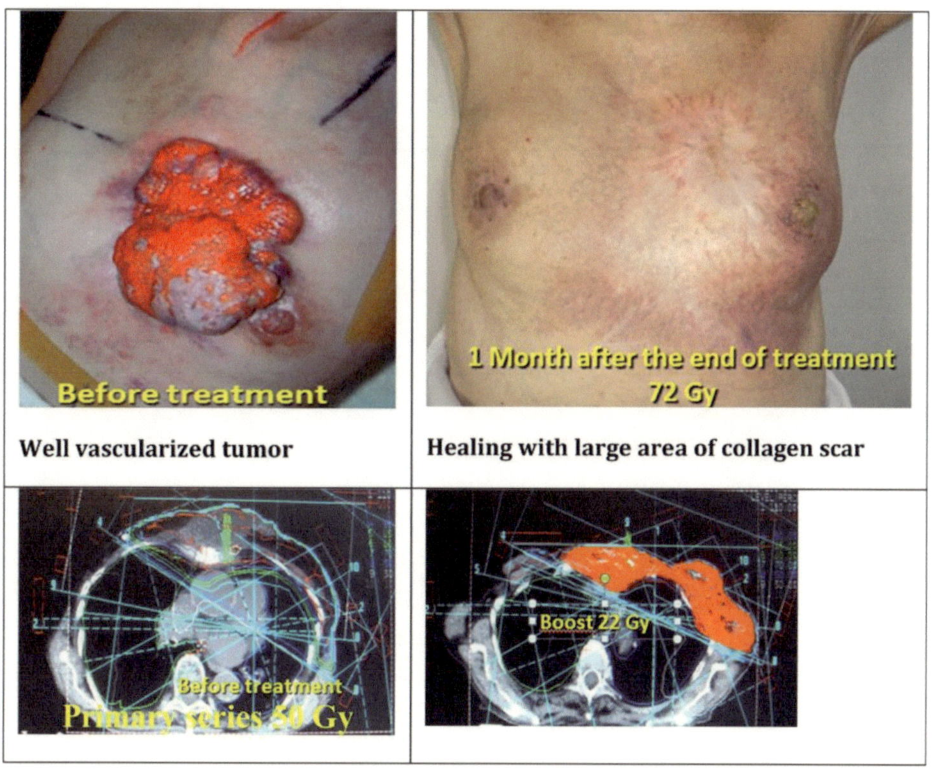

Figure 11.
The clinical case of a local advanced breast cancer with sternal infiltration and internal mammary chain lymph node involvement before and after high dose radiotherapy. Upper line: Clinical response to a high total dose of 72 Gy. Lower line: (left) in the primary series a total dose of 50 Gy in 25 fractions and (right) an additional boost of 22 Gy in 2 Gy fractionation was applied.

This case demonstrates the "remodeling" ability that exists in healthy tissues surrounding the tumor bed. In this case, the healing action was completed by macrophages and fibroblasts present at this level. The action of fibroblasts has contributed to the collagen formation process to be present and to make possible "remodeling" at this level of all the structures initially involved: skin, ribs, pericardium, sternum, etc. Visible is the presence of an extensive area of collagen in the extensive scar.

In the healing process, the role of macrophages was the removal of damaged tumor cells by the double-strand lesion at the level of tumor DNA. There was no pulmonary fibrosis that usually accompanies post-radiotherapy healing [6].

9.4 Remodeling of bone metastases

Radiotherapy is the most important treatment for bone metastases. Long-term local control of the disease is possible.

In **Figure 12** we present a patient treated over years with bone metastases throughout the skeleton and taking advantage of radiotherapy with standard doses of 2 Gy per fraction and an accumulated total dose of 676 Gy to achieve tumor control. A survival of almost four years was possible. The primary tumor in the breast was treated by surgery followed by adjuvant chest wall radiotherapy in 1979. The first bone metastasis was irradiated in 8/1993 and the last palliative radiotherapy was applied in 5/1997 [6].

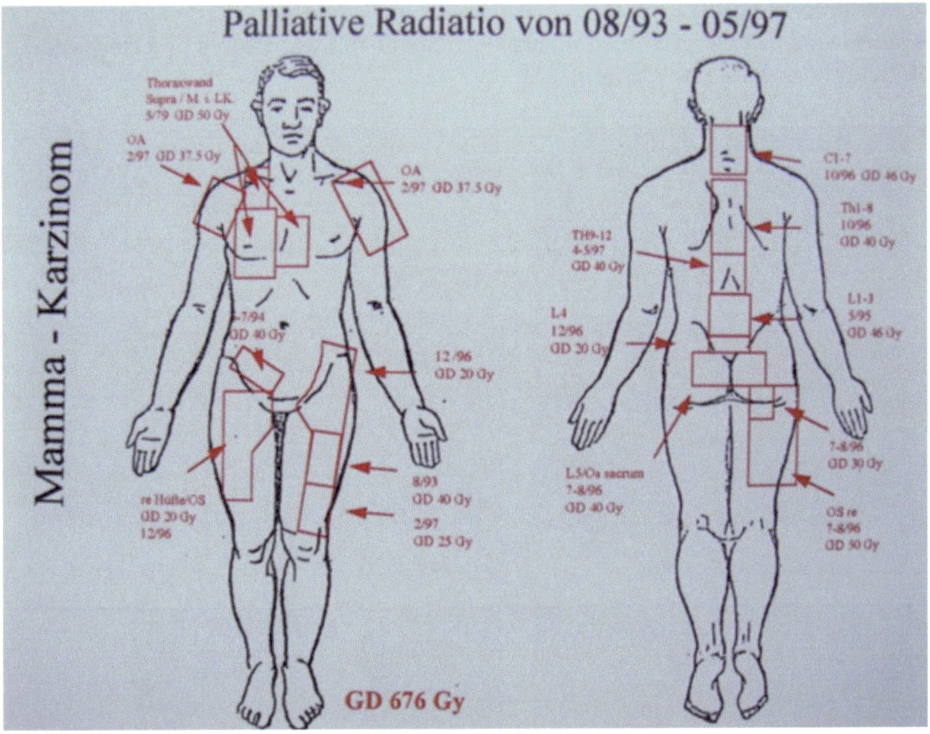

Figure 12.
Irradiated regions of the bone skeleton in a patient with a breast tumor who survived 4 years with radiation therapy.

9.4.1 Bone metastasis and remodeling processes in the extracellular matrix

Cellular processes at the level of bone metastasis: after homing of tumor cells endosteal, the tumor cells release endothelin, which, through its appropriate

DOI: http://dx.doi.org/10.5772/intechopen.102732

receptors, interact with osteoblasts to stimulate their proliferation. This leads to the formation of new bone and growth, but such bone is weak and prone to fracture. Activated osteoblasts release receptor activator, that signals the proliferation and maturation of osteoclasts. They stimulate macrophages to produce pro-inflammatory cytokines and prostaglandins, which induce pain by binding to their receptors on sensory neurons.

9.4.2 Remodeling is facilitated by initiating the radiotherapy of bone metastasis

With the location of the tumor cell in the bone, begins the process of damaging its compact structure. Stromal and pro-inflammatory cells recruited by tumor cells such as macrophages, neutrophils, T cells, and mastoid cells produce and release many mediators that act on osteoblasts, osteoclasts, and nerve endings at this level. The most important is the endothelin which initiates the process of stimulating osteoblasts that releases the so-called RANKL which is an activator that initiates the maturation and proliferation of the osteoclasts. Osteoclasts promote demineralization, destruction, and bone lysis. They stimulate macrophages to produce pro-inflammatory cytokines (TNF-alpha, IL-ß, and IL6) and pain-inducing prostaglandins by binding them to receptors in neuronal sensors (**Figure 13**).

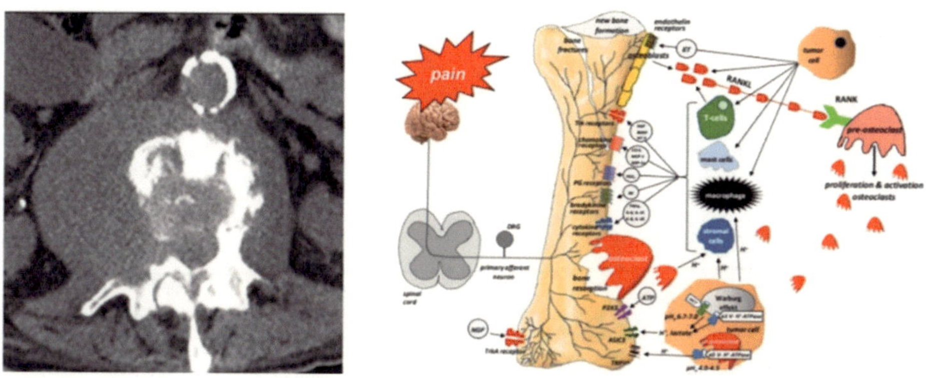

Figure 13.
Left: Bone metastasis with the destruction of the vertebra (non-small cell lung cancer) and with the invasion of the paravertebral muscle (treated at an oncology center with a single fraction of 8 Gy). Subsequently, the patient died with only this distant metastasis. Right: Mechanisms from the initiation of bone metastasis (activation of osteoclast) followed by osteolysis and the mechanism of central pain transmission [11].

All therapeutic interventions must be individualized and directed in order to reduce pain so that an improvement in the quality of life should be achieved, and thus, facilitate to prolongation of life with longer survival. Only by reducing pain will not be achieved an improvement in survival, this action must also be sustained by total destruction of the tumor itself. A single dose of 8 Gy applied to a single bone metastasis to a vertebral body will bring a reduction in pain, but the patient will not have a longer survival if the metastasis itself is not destroyed, which with only 8 Gy cannot be achieved. The possible right treatment could be the application of an initial dose of 8 Gy, which makes it possible to reduce pain and continue irradiation with fractional doses of 2 or 3 Gy up to a total dose equivalent to 40 Gy at the level of the vertebral body, a dose that also allows the destruction of tumor cells.

This kind of "palliation" is recommended in the guidelines and applied in clinical activity. The misunderstanding of the differentiated action of high single doses can lead only to pain control (success rate of 45%) but only for lasting few days. "Improved quality of life for only a few days" is paid for by subsequent death, due to the insufficient dose applied to control the tumor itself for years.

Bone remodeling is a continuous process initiated by the action of radiotherapy or/and bisphosphonate on osteoclasts and thus allows osteoblasts to initiate the remodeling phase with bone formation, especially at the periosteum and endosteum level. Here it should be remembered the importance of the action of the macrophage at this level called **osteomacs** which has the most important role in the "remodeling" of the bone. It should be remembered that in general the skeletal system has the capacity to maintain the stability and functional malleability of the entire bone system and that annually 10% of the bone system is renewed. So, in 10 years we take advantage of a "physiological" remodeling and maintenance of our entire bone system.

Tanaka et al. [12] reported a combined treatment with zoledronic acid and fractional radiotherapy applied to metastasis in a vertebral body, that affected the stability of the spine. The clinical result of this combined treatment in which the total dose in that fractionation allowed to stop the action of osteoclasts and initiate **osteomacs activity** with the result of "remodeling" and healing of the vertebral body using the initial matrix of the vertebral body it is shown in **Figure 14** [6].

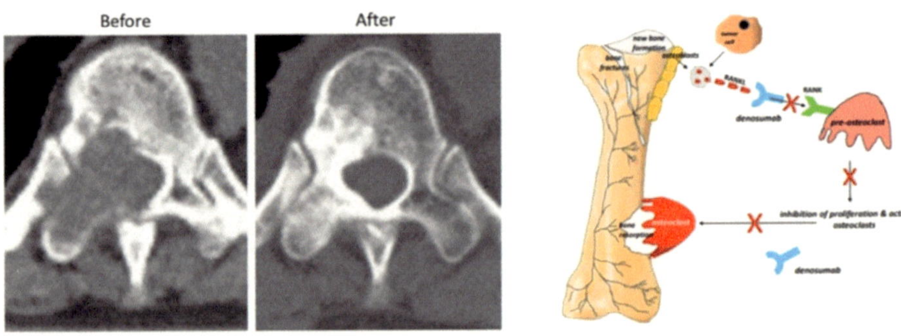

Figure 14.
Left: Complete remodeling of vertebral metastasis. Improvement of osteolytic metastasis from a vertebral body after administration of zoledronic acid and external radiotherapy with 28 Gy in seven fractions [12]. Right: The role of the RANKL/RANK system and the mechanism of action of Denosumab in bone pain. X = stop [11].

9.4.3 Remodeling of multiple bone metastasis with bone destruction

Radiation therapy of multiple bone metastases and complete destruction of the right coxo-femoral joint of breast cancer in the bone pelvis is presented. Restitutio ad integrum of all bone metastases and especially of the right coxo-femoral joint with the restoration of the acetabulum was possible.

Patients with multiple pelvic bones metastases, like the one presented below, could profit from whole pelvic bone radiotherapy. The patient was irradiated with a 2 Gy daily fraction to a total dose of 40 Gy. The protection of organs at risk as the bladder, small bowel, rectum, and sigmoid was possible. Multiple lytic bone lesions and complete destruction of the acetabulum were present. Two years later all bone lesions and the acetabulum destruction were in complete restitution, as shown in the **Figure 15** [6].

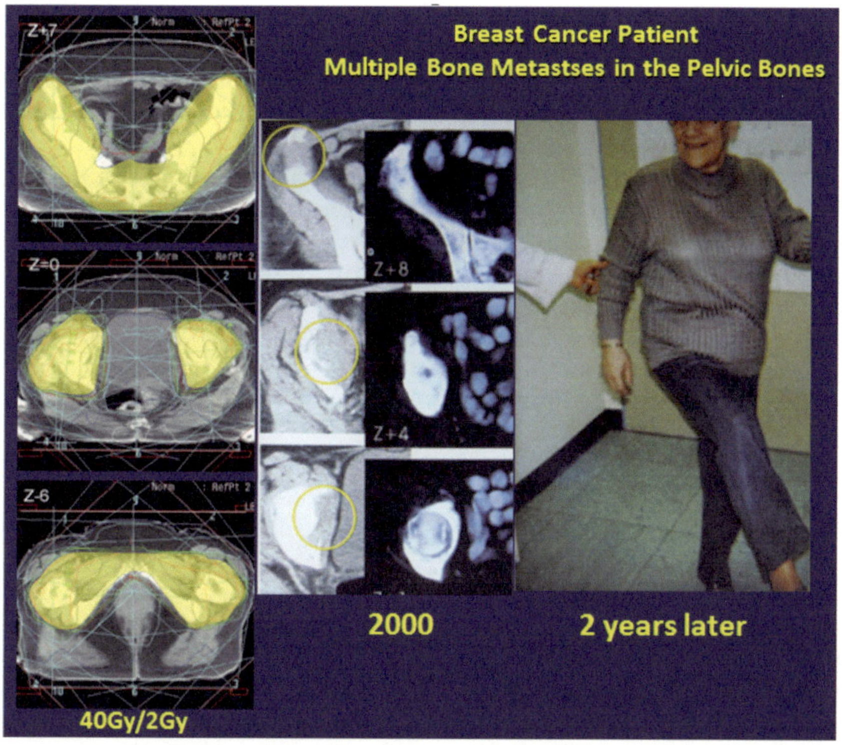

Figure 15.
Dose distribution of the whole pelvic bone radiotherapy (left side), bone reconstruction after radiotherapy (middle), and clinical situation 2 years later (right side).

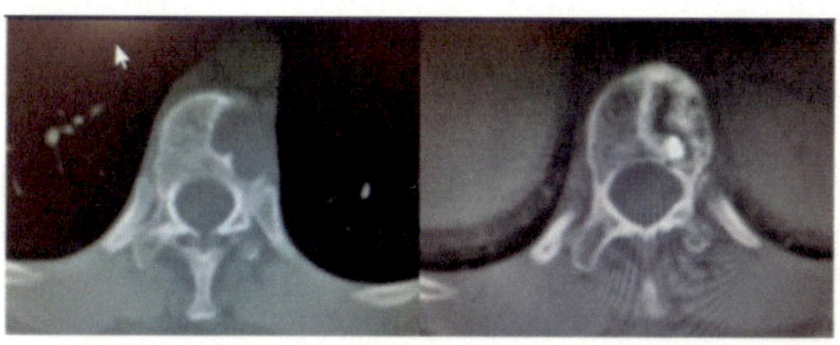

Before ***(left)*** *and after radiotherapy* ***(right)*** *of the metastatic vertebra with the restoration of the initial shape of the vertebral body.*

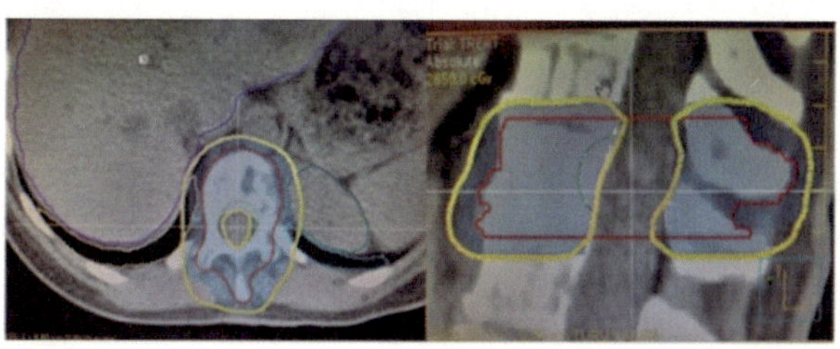

Irradiation plane of the thoracic vertebra T11 with the spinal cord protection
Dose applied: 30 Gy in 10 fractions.

Figure 16.
Remodeling at the vertebral body, evolution, and irradiation plan of a vertebral body metastasis.

9.4.4 Remodeling of vertebral metastases

Restoration of the shape of the thoracic vertebra after surgery and postoperative radiotherapy of bone metastasis of breast cancer in the thoracic spine at the level of T11 is shown in **Figure 16**.

In the previous images can be observed osteolysis produced by tumor cells located in the vertebral body at the beginning endosteal, which activates the osteoclasts and starts the destruction of the periosteum, compromising completely the stability of the vertebrae. In this case, 10 fractions of 3 Gy were applied, which made it possible to initiate the remodeling process and through the action of osteomacs and osteoblasts appeared "the new" remodeled bone that followed exactly the initial matrix of the vertebral body, being thus possible an ad integrum reconstruction of the final shape of the vertebral body after radiotherapy [6].

10. Conclusion and final remarks

The progress in radiotherapy is a result of improved imaging methods (CT, MRI, PET/CT) and as well as developed planning and dose delivery methods as VMAT, Rapid Arc, and Tomotherapy, techniques based on individually defined target volumes. Optimal dose delivery to CTV and GTV and limited dose delivery to organs at risk as lung parenchyma, brachial plexus, myocardial tissue, and axillary vessels is now possible. Higher tumor control rates with less acute and late side effects make now possible the improvement of the quality of life [5]. Remodeling of ECM of TME should be a reality if adequate irradiation technique and proper fractionation and the total dose are optimally selected.

Radiotherapy is an integral modality of cancer treatment. Changes in TME produced by therapy have fundamental consequences and make possible the cure of cancer. These processes are spatially and temporally regulated to preserve the homeostasis of tissues and involve the interplay of different cell types. Tissue homeostasis is maintained by REMODELING of BASEMENT MEMBRANE as was noted in many of the cases presented in this chapter. Different compartments of TME are closely related to and contribute not only to tumor progression but also to its response to treatment.

We should not forget that TME is affected by different therapeutic modalities. Changes in TME make possible: reduced tumor burden, improvement of oxygenation by normalization of the vasculature, reduced radio resistance, and improvement of the access of chemotherapy and immunotherapy to the tumor.

ECM remodeling is essential and tightly regulates physiological processes in development and in restoring tissue homeostasis during wound repair.

Knowledge regarding ECM dysregulation in the design of anticancer therapy is necessary. With the advances and interdisciplinary integration, progress in an anticancer strategy targeting TME and ECM components could improve the quality of life of cancer patients.

Author details

Ion Christian Chiricuta
AMETHYST Radiotherapy Center, Otopeni, Romania

*Address all correspondence to: kirikuta@gmx.de

References

[1] Henke E, Nandigama R, Ergun S. Extracellular matrix in the tumor microenvironment and its impact on cancer therapy. Frontiers in Molecular Biosciences. 2020;**6**:160. DOI: 10.3389/fmolb.2019.00160

[2] Farnsworth RH, Lackermann M, Achen MG, Stacker SA. Vascular remodeling in cancer. Oncogene. 2014;**33**:3496-3505. DOI: 10.1038/onc.2013.304

[3] Potiron V, Clement-Colmou K, Jouglar E, Petri M, Chiavassa S, Delpon G, et al. Tumor vasculature remodeling by radiation therapy increases doxorubicin distribution and efficacy. Cancer Letters. 2019;**457**:1-9. DOI: 10.1016/j.canlet.2019.05.005

[4] Richter E, Bohndorf W. Target volume determination with CT in pharynx and larynx tumors. Radiotherapy and Oncology. 1986;**162**:162-170

[5] Jin GH, Chen LX, Deng XW, Liu XW, Huang Y, Huang XB. A comparative dosimetric study for treating left-sided breast cancer for small breast size using five different radiotherapy techniques: Conventional tangential field, field-in-field, tangential-IMRT, multi-beam IMRT and VMAT. Radiation Oncology. 2013;**8**:89. DOI: 10.1186/1748-717X-8-89

[6] Chiricuta IC. New language and old problems in breast cancer radiotherapy. Chirurgia (Buc). 2017;**112**(4):394-402

[7] Bentzen SM. Preventing or reducing late side effects of radiation therapy: Radiobiology meets molecular pathology. Nature Reviews. 2006;**6**:703-713. DOI: 10.1038/nrc1950

[8] Poltavets V, Kochelkova M, Pitson M, Samuel MS. The role of extracellular matrix and its cell regulators in cancer cells plasticity. Frontiers in Oncology. 2018;**431**:1-19. DOI: 10.3389/fonc.2018.00431

[9] Maynard J. How Wounds Heal: The Four Main Phases of Wound Healing. Shield Health Care; 2015

[10] Lali FV, Metcalfe AD. The role of angiogenesis in wound healing, scarring and tissue regeneration. PMFA News. 2014;**2**(1):1-4. Available from: www.pmfanews.com

[11] Zajaczkowska R, Kocot-Kepska M, Leppert W, Wordliczek J. Bone pain in cancer patients: Mechanisms and current treatment. International Journal of Molecular Sciences. 2019;**20**(23):6047. DOI: 10.3390/ijms20236047

[12] Tanaka H, Makita CH, Manabe Y, Kajima M, Matsuyama K, Matsuo M. Radiation therapy combined with bone-modifying agents ameliorates local control of osteolytic bone metastases in breast cancer. Journal of Radiation Research. 2020;**61**(3):494-498. DOI: 10.1093/jrr/rraa020

Section 2

Dosimetry

Chapter 6

Dosimetry Audit in Modern Radiotherapy

Katia Manolova Sergieva

Abstract

The clinical specialty of radiotherapy is an essential part of the multidisciplinary process of treatment of malignant neoplasms. Modern radiotherapy is a very complex process of treatment planning and delivery of radiation dose. Radiotherapy reached a very high degree of complexity and sophistication and expected to represent an added value for the cancer patients in terms of clinical outcomes and improved radiation protection. The concept of verifying the realized dose in the medical applications of ionizing radiation was introduced in the early 20th century shortly after the first application of X-rays for the treatment of cancer. Dosimetry audit identify areas for improvement and provide confidence in safety and efficacy, which are essential to creating a clinical environment of continuous development and improvement. Over the years, the audits have contributed to good dosimetry practice and accuracy of dose measurements in modern radiotherapy. Dosimetry audit ensures, that the correct therapeutic dose is delivered to the patients undergoing radiotherapy and play a key role in activities to create a good radiation protection and safety culture. Patient safety is of paramount importance to medical staff in radiotherapy centers and safety considerations are an element in all aspects of the day-to-day clinical activities.

Keywords: modern radiotherapy, clinical audit, dosimetry audit, radiation dosimetry measurements, radiophotoluminescent dosimeters (RPLD), quality assurance, quality managemnet

1. Introduction

The clinical specialty of radiotherapy is an essential part of the multidisciplinary process of treatment of malignant neoplasms. Moreover, oncological diseases are and will continue to be a growing health - social and socio - economic problem nationally and globally in the coming decades. The development of the clinical method of radiotherapy is based on advances in nuclear and information technology. In recent years, dramatic and I would say revolutionary changes have taken place in connection with the introduction into routine practice of a number of new methods and radiotherapy techniques for delivering of the therapeutic dose. All these innovations, set the requirements for the development of precise and clear rules, criteria and standards for the quality of the radiotherapy process as well as for conducting a regular dosimetric quality audit. Clinical audit is defined as a process of quality improvement that seeks to improve patient care and outcomes by systematically reviewing the clinical activity performed against certain formulated criteria [1].

The quality audit in radiotherapy is an independent review of the quality assurance programs, which is ideally external to the process or part of the process being audited, ie. it is performed through independent procedures and by independent staff, who are not responsible for the performance of the activities, that are the subject of the audit.

The purpose of the introduction and development of the concept of external audit in the radiotherapy is to create and maintain a consistently high quality of the treatment method. The external audit ensures, that the clinical requirements for the quality of radiotherapy are met to achieve optimal treatment in terms of maximizing the likelihood of tumor control, while maintaining low normal tissue damage within clinically acceptable levels. As part of this, the implementation of a quality assurance program will minimize errors and incidents. Most countries seek to establish transparent quality management systems in health care for a number of reasons - professional, social, financial and political. The main goal of this form of quality assurance (QA) is to improve patient care with the intention of maximizing the effect of clinical activities, minimizing harm to the individual and society as a whole.

Achieving high quality in clinical practice in general and in radiation therapy in particular is a fundamental goal. The effectiveness of the clinical method of radiotherapy depends on the exact reproducibility of the patient's position, the technical parameters of the irradiation systems and the exact dosimetric calibration of the used photon or electron beams of radiation, which are subject to international standards. The technical achievements and the conducted clinical studies impose the need of quality control programs and respectively external dosimetric audit of the radiation therapy process. This has led to the development and publication of a large number of international recommendations. The aim is to provide reliable, effective and precise radiation therapy. One of the key element is the organization and conducting of dosimetry audit in modern radiation therapy.

2. Modern radiotherapy

Cancer is a leading cause of death worldwide, accounting for nearly 10 million deaths in 2020. The most common in 2020 (in terms of new cases of cancer) are: breast (2.26 million cases); lung (2.21 million cases); colon and rectum (1.93 million cases); prostate (1.41 million cases); skin (non-melanoma) (1.20 million cases) and stomach (1.09 million cases) [2]. Radiotherapy is recognized as an essential element of an effective cancer care program throughout the world. It is vital component of the treatment of cancer for many years. Aproximatelly half of all cancer patients requiring a radiotherapy in some time of their deceases. Abdel-Wahab et al. [3], Barton et al. [4], and Atun et al. [5], argue, that radiotherapy is a critical and cost-effective component of a comprehensive cancer control plan [6].

Modern radiotherapy is a very complex process of treatment planning and delivery of radiation dose. Today, radiotherapy encompasses a lot of steps from clinical evaluation to posttreatment follow-up. The clinical process of modern radiation therapy starts with a therapeutic decision at the first appointment with cancer patient, where the radiation oncologist prescribes the radiotherapy treatment. Then the immobilization of patient is performed, which be adopted during treatment. A computerized tomography (CT) scan of the patient is acquired for delineations of the planning target volumes (PTV) and the organs-at-risk (OARs). The CT images may be fusion with other imaging modalities such as magnetic resonance imaging (MRI) and positron emission tomography (PET) for the precise determination of PTV and OARs. A treatment plan is created on a treatment planning system (TPS) based on the outlined structures and on the dose prescription to the PTV and tolerance dose criteria to the OARs. A pre-treatment quality assurance (QA) verification of the treatment plan has been performed after its evaluation and approving by the radiation oncologist. Image guided radiation therapy (IGRT) modality is using to check patient positioning before each treatment.

In recent years, radiotherapy has been advancing toward achieving a higher cure rate with a higher therapeutic dose and minimum side-effects. This has been possible through the development of high-performance and highprecision radiotherapy techniques and by applying cutting-edge medical technologies [7].

Modern radiotherapy reached a very high degree of complexity and sophistication and expected to represent an added value for the cancer patients in terms of clinical outcomes and improved radiation protection.

In 2016, IAEA published a new guidance document titled: Accuracy Requirements and Uncertainties in Radiotherapy [8]. All forms of radiotherapy should be applied as accurately as reasonably achievable with technical and biological factors being considered, but that regular independent dosimetry audit be conducted using postal (remote) or on-site visits [9].

3. History of dosimetry audit

The concept of verifying the realized dose in the medical applications of ionizing radiation was introduced in the early 20th century shortly after the first application of X-rays for the treatment of cancer.

Initially, in order to adequately assess the daily fraction that would be prescribed to patients, doctors irradiated their own hands to observe a skin reaction - "dose of erythema".

In 1925, the Swedish physicist R. Sievert [10] created a circulating physical department to standardize the Roentgen radiation (X-rays) used in oncology therapy in his country. The department found some unreliable dosimeters and identified the need for better protective equipment for X-ray personnel. At the same time, the data collected from the measurements of the dosimetric value - Percent Depth Dose (PDD) were used as reference values for the technical equipment used for clinical purposes at that time.

Another documented example of an early dosimetry audit was found in Poland, following Marie Curie's idea that a Laboratory for measuring the dose of X-rays and the radioactive isotope radium used in hospitals at the time should be opened. The laboratory for dosimetry measurements was founded in 1936 [10].

The dosimety laboratory in the International Atomic Energy Agency (IAEA) was established in the early 1960s to organize and conduct dosimetry audits for radiotherapy centers worldwide and to ensure international consistency in radiation dosimetry. The first pilot postal comparison of the radiation dose between different radiotherapy centers was organized by the IAEA in the period 1965–1966 as a joint project with the World Health Organization (WHO).

4. The essence of dosimetry audit

Dosimetry audit (DA) is a tool for quality improvement. It can be defined as a systematic and critical analysis of the quality of the dosimetry activities performed in specific radiotherapy center. The dosimetry audit includes an assessment of data, documents and resources in order to verify the performed clinical dosimetry activity against the adopted international standards of good practice. The essence of the dosimetry audit can be summarized as:

- Improving the quality and organization of the dosimetry activities.
- Further professional training of medical physicists.
- Increasing the efficiency and safety of the radiotherapy.
- Improving the quality of the overall radiotherapy process.
- Promoting the efficient use of available resources.

The results of the dosimetry audit inform the staff about the main elements of the quality and the weaknesses of the dosimetry activities carried out, comparing the audited dosimetric practice with the standards for good clinical radiation dosimetry. Dosimetry audit identify areas for improvement and provide confidence in safety and efficacy, which are essential to creating a clinical environment of continuous development and improvement.

One of the main risks for patients undergoing radiation therapy is the delivery of a dosimetry inaccurate therapeutic dose during radiation therapy sessions. Dosimetry inaccuracies directly reflect on tumor control, cancer treatment and toxicity affected the survival, and quality of life of cancer patients. The differences between the prescribed and delivered dose directly affect the clinical outcomes. The precision of the therapeutic method of radiation therapy is mainly related to the high degree of accuracy of the radiation dose applied during the treatment of patients.

Dosimetry audit is a partial audit and related to the quality assurance procedures in the field of the performed dosimetry activities in a specific radiotherapy center and namely [11–13]:

- Quality tool that improves the accuracy of clinical radistion dosimetry.
- Conducted on a voluntary basis, but each radiotherapy center must initiate it itself.
- DA is a "second opinion", regardless of the specific treatment center regarding the performed clinical dosimetry - procedures, protocols, measuring instruments, etc.
- Identifies gaps in procedures and methods used as well as errors in routine practice.
- Identifying and understanding of errors leads to improved quality in general in the clinical activities of specific radiotherapy center.
- Illustrates the good dosimetry practice in the field of radiation clinical dosimetry based on world standards.
- Contributes to the avoidance of accidents and omissions in the daily radiotherapy activity.
- DA is confidential.
- DA leads to the exchange of knowledge, skills, information and competence.

Dosimetry audit is proactive, ie. consists in reviewing the current clinical dosimetry in order to improve its quality. It is organized and conducted remotely, ie. It is (remote audit).

Dosimetry audit worldwide are organized in different ways, often for geographical, economic or political reasons, but mainly check the fundamental value - the absorbed dose in reference conditions, ie. so-called - beam output [12]. The measurement of the value of the absorbed dose in the so-called reference conditions i.e. beam output is the most fundamental measurement that confirms whether the therapeutic system generating ionizing radiation and used for radiotherapy is properly calibrated [14].

The existence of an error in the calibration of the radiation beams leads to the creation of a systemic error in the treatment of each individual patient, which in turn leads to systemic differences in the results of the conducted radiation therapy.

DA is a key component in quality management in radiotherapy and plays an important role in the safe application and use of new methods and techniques of radiotherapy [15, 16].

5. Types of dosimetry audit

The International Atomic Energy Agency (IAEA) as the founder of the idea of dosimetry audit and main organizator of the program for postal dosimetryc audit with thermoluminescent dosimeters (TLDs) and radiophotoluminescent dosimeters (RPLDs) for nearly fifty years has identified the following types [17] (See **Figure 1**).

Level	Tasks	Dosimetry equipment	Phantom
Level 1	Verification of the photon and electron beam output under reference conditions	**R**[(1)]: TLD, OSLD, RPLD Alanine **O**[(1)]: Ion chamber, 2D & 3D Array, TLD, OSLD, RPLD, Alanine	Water Geometric/solid
Level 2	Verification of the photon and electron beam relative dosimetry parameters under non-reference conditions on- and off-central axis	**R**: TLD, OSLD, RPLD, Alanine, films, diodes **O**: Ion chamber, 2D & 3D Array, films, diodes, TLD, OSLD, RPLD, Alanine	Water Geometric/solid
Level 3	Verification of complex dosimetry parameters using geometric / rectilinear phantom or anthropomorphic phantom. Treatment planning system (TPS) dose calculations are compared to audit measurements.	**R**: TLD, OSLD, RPLD Alanine, films, diodes, 2D & 3D Array **O**: Ion chamber, 2D & 3D Array, films, diodes, TLD, OSLD, RPLD, Alanine	Water Geometric/solid Anthropomorphic
Level 4	Verification of advanced treatment modalities, e.g. IMRT, VMAT, SRS, SRT, using an end-to-end anthropomorphic phantom that approximates a patient treatment, including targets, organs at risk and heterogeneities.	**R**: TLD, OSLD, RPLD, Alanine, films, diodes, 3D dosimeters (e.g. polymer, PRESAGE, Fricke gels) **O**: Ion chamber, 2D & 3D Array, films, diodes, TLD, OSLD, RPLD, Alanine, 3D dosimeters (e.g. polymer, PRESAGE, Fricke gels)	Anthropomorphic

[(1)] **R**: Remote audits, **O**: On-site audits

Figure 1.
IAEA classification of different types dosimetry audits [17].

6. Current status of dosimetry audit in the member countries of the european federation of organizations for medical physics (EFOMP)

The European Union has issued a new directive on the use of ionizing radiation for medical purposes 2013/58 / EURATOM, which entered into force in 2014 [18]. The new Directive updates the basic standards for radiation protection in clinical and professional settings, emphasizes clinical audits, reinforces their importance for quality improvement and recommends, that Member States ensure that dosimetry audits are carried out in accordance with national audit procedures.

A clinical audit is defined as "a systematic review or review of medical radiological procedures that seeks to improve the quality and outcome of patient care through a structured review in which medical radiological practices, procedures and outcomes are performed against established standards for good medical radiological procedures. procedures, changing practices where appropriate and applying new standards if necessary."

Dosimetry audits are one of the main measures introduced to ensure the safety of patients undergoing radiotherapy. The international organizations conducting clinical trials set as a condition for participation the results of the dosimeter audit in order to evaluate the clinical dosimetry in the specific radiotherapy center, with it participated in the clinical trial [19]. In this way, dosimetry quality assurance (QA) and quality control (QC) are doubled as a tool in the fine-tuning used in clinical trial technology [20].

Performing an external dosimetry audit is an expensive procedure that requires special knowledge, skills, actions, time and effort. In some countries, basic safety standards require regular dosimetric audits with different requirements and frequencies.

The audit documentation of radiotherapy centers participating in an international clinical trial is not always easy to obtain and analyze because it is heterogeneous in terms of the type and frequency of dosimetric audit and is different for different centers and countries in Europe.

All this is the basis of the European Federation of Organizations for Medical Physics (EFOMP) to initiate a survey to determine what kind of audit, clinical or dosimetric, is required by law in different European countries, what role the medical physicist plays and to get a general idea for the regulations and practices regarding the quality assurance and quality control of the radiotherapy equipment.

EFOMP is developing a questionnaire in order to obtain the necessary information on the general requirements and standards for organizing and conducting dosimetric audit, quality assurance of dosimetric activity and periodic dosimetric inspections in EU countries at the end of 2019. The questions are addressed to the community of medical physicists to assess the regulatory status of dosimetric audits performed in radiotherapy centers.

The questionnaire was sent to 33 National Member Organizations (NMOs) in November 2019 (at the time of the survey's dissemination, 33 NMOs were part of EFOMP). The results were obtained in the period December 2019–March 2020.

The first section of the questionnaire refers to the requirements for conducting periodic dosimetric audits in radiotherapy centers in Europe, the subject (auditor) performing the audit according to national legislation, as well as the source of the auditor (internal / external).

19 NMOs (58%) of the 33 EFOM members replied to the questionnaire. Of these, 14 are EU Member States (54%) and 5 are non-EU (46%).

In eleven European countries (11/19 NMOs), 9 EU members and 2 non-EU countries, national regulations require regular dosimetric audits to be carried out in radiotherapy centers (See **Figure 2**).

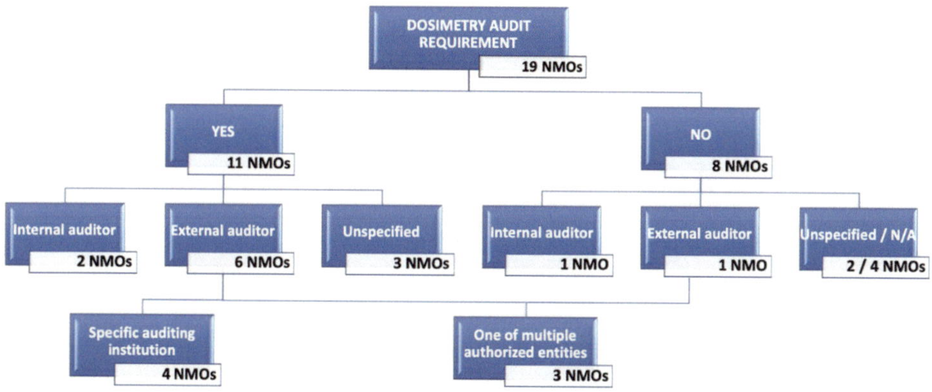

Figure 2.
Dosimetric audit requirements according to the NMO responses [20].

Dosimetry audits are performed as follows: by external auditors in (6/11 NMOs), by internal auditors (2/11 NMOs) and by an unspecified auditor in (3/11 NMOs). 42% (8/19 NMOs), of which 5 EU members and 3 non-EU countries state that the requirements for conducting a dosimetric audit are not regulated at national level.

Only 11 NMOs report that national regulations require regular dosimetric audits of radiotherapy centers, but only 6 European countries state that there are well-established procedures that must be followed for an audit to be valid. Dosimetric audit is of great interest to EFOMP and is given great importance in Council Directive 2013/59 / EURATOM. Overall, the EFOMP study shows significant heterogeneity in national policies on the dosimetric audit program of radiotherapy centers.

Dosimetric audits were conducted in only 58% of the countries (NMOs) that participated in the survey organized and conducted by EFOMP in November 2019, although the deadline for transposition of the European Directive 2013/59 / EURATOM into national legislations is the end of 2019.

7. Radiophotoluminescent dosimeters (RPLDs)

The physical phenomenon of photoluminescence is the basis for the detection of ionizing radiation with radiophotoluminescent dosimeters. Radiophotoluminescence as a phenomenon shows that some materials, after irradiation with sources of ionizing radiation, begin to luminesce under illumination with ultraviolet (UV) light and the luminescent light is proportional to the dose they were irradiated [21] (See **Figures 3** and **4**).

This effect was used to create radiophotoluminescent (RFL) dosimeters, which are alumina-phosphate glasses, activated with silver and synthesized by a special technology that used the effect of photoluminescence.

In 1949, the RPL phenomenon was first discovered and applied for measuring the dose in the event of a radiation accident. The magnitude of the radiation dose ranged from 0.1 to 1 Gy [22]. At that time, there were still some problems with glass surface contamination and measuring the RPL signal became a technical challenge. Later, the ability to register ionizing radiation was drastically improved by changing the chemical composition of the glass used. Thus, the measurement range is from 0.1 mGy to 10 Gy [23].

Radiophotoluminescent dosimeters are an accumulative type of dosimeter. They work on the principle of the phenomenon of radiophotoluminescence, which is

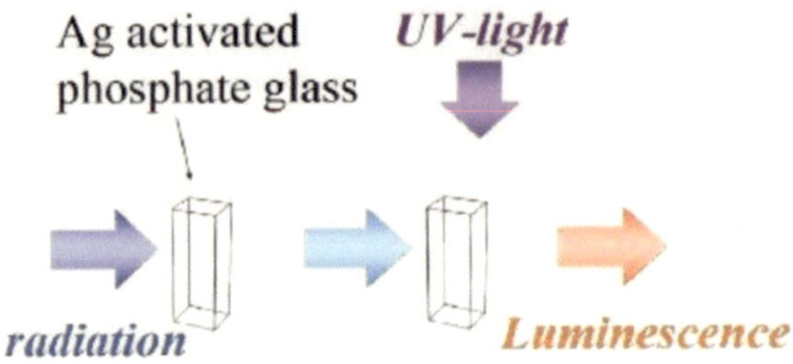

Figure 3.
Schematic representation of the RPL process in phosphate glass doped with silver Ag+ ions [21].

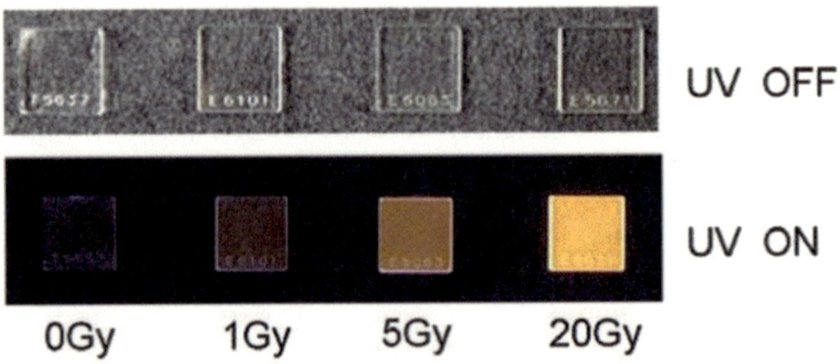

Figure 4.
The amount of luminescent light is proportional to the radiation dose [21].

observed in some solids. RPLDs are made of silver-activated phosphate glass and are shaped like small glass rods (See **Figure 5**).

The glass rods are 12 mm long and 1.5 mm in diameter. Each glass rod has an identification number engraved on one end. The sensitive area of the dosimeter is 6 mm long. When irradiated with ionizing radiation, stable luminescent centers are formed in the silver ions - positive and negative. The measurement of the absorbed dose is performed by optical excitation of the dosimeter with a laser emitting ultraviolet light [21]. The first RPLD was produced in 1949 [22]. Significant technological improvements have been made over time, including the accuracy and reliability of their measurement [23]. They are currently one of the best solid state dosimeters [21].

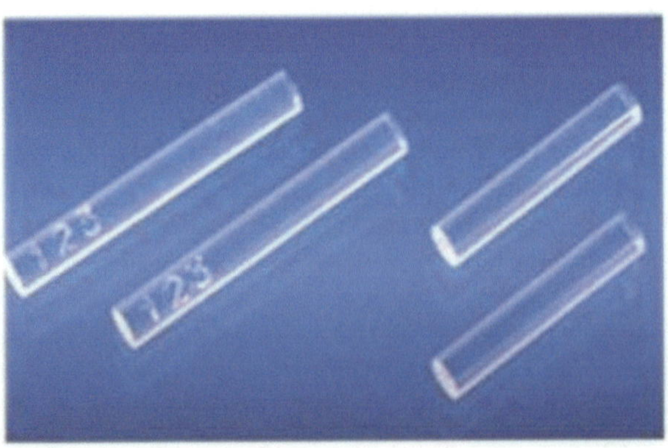

Figure 5.
General type of radiophotoluminescent dosimeters (RPLDs) – glass rods.

Today, the production of RPL dosimetry is advancing remarkably thanks to modern electronics and is well accepted as a solid-state, passive dosimeter operating in the range of 10μGy to 10 Gy, using a pulsed laser beam of UV light. Radiophotoluminescence dosimeters (RPLD) as a new type of solid state dosimeters are used in radiation dosimetry for radiotherapy in the last two decades.

8. Dosimety audit with radiophotoluminescent dosimeters (RPLDs) in reference conditions

The dosimetry system based on radiophotoluminescent dosimeters (RPLDs) is the Ace Dosimetry System, consisting of GD-302 M glass rods and an FDG-1000 reader from Asahi Techno Glass Corporation (ATG). It is used in IAEA Dosimetry Laboaratory (See **Figure 6**).

The glass rods are made of silver-activated phosphate glass. They are 12 mm long and 1.5 mm in diameter. Each glass rod has an identification number engraved on one end. The sensitive area of the dosimeter is 6 mm long. The glass rods are placed in specially made waterproof capsules. Each capsule with a glass rod already placed in it can be considered as an *RPLD Dosimeter* (See **Figure 7**). The capsules, model M5001 produced by MISATO Precision Inc., is made of high density polyethylene (HDPE, Nipolon Hard 2000, Tosoh Corporation, Japan). It consists of a container with approximate cylindrical symmetry and with an internal 12.1-mm-long cylindrical cavity of 1.8 mm of diameter [24].

The dosimetry audit with RPLDs is the newest form of the audit offering as a service by IAEA Dosimetry Laboratory to the Member States. The participants

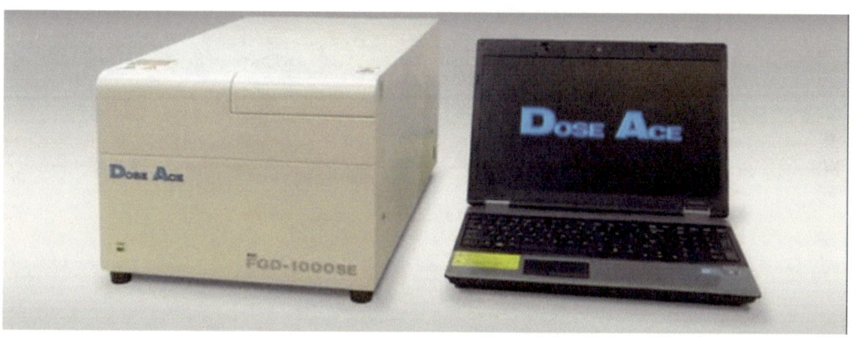

Figure 6.
Dose Ace dosimetry system consisting of GD-302 M glass rods and an FGD-1000 reader/analyzer from the Japanese Asahi Techno Glass Corporation (ATG).

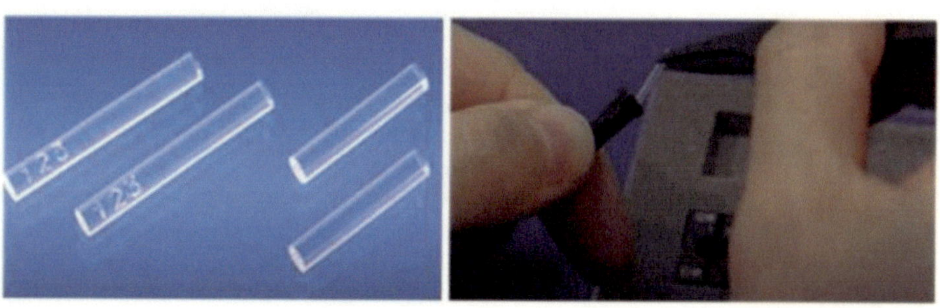

Figure 7.
Glass rods on the left and waterproof capsule on the right.

(radiotherapy centers) should to irradiate the RPLDs in a water phantom using an IAEA standard holder in reference conditions: S = 10x10 cm field size, 10 cm depth in water phantom and nominal Source Surface Distance (SSD) or Source Axis Distance (SAD) of 100 cm used clinically.

Each capsule has an ID number and a bar code. The sensitive area is also marked on the capsule to allow precise positioning (See **Figure 8**).

The purpose of the dosimetric audit is to perform the measurements specified in the instruction in the same conditions under which the patients are irradiated on daily basis (See **Figure 9**).

The irradiation procedure of RPLDs includes the following steps according to the IAEA instruction sheet [25, 26]:

I. Preparation of beam, phantom and hoder for irradiation of RPLDs.

1. Assemble the holder (**Figure 10**).

2. Place the holder in a water tank on the treatment table (**Figure 11**).

3. Set the therapy unit for a vertical beam, with a 10 cm x 10 cm field size (**Figure 11**).

4. Align the holder tube with the central axis of the beam (**Figure 11**).

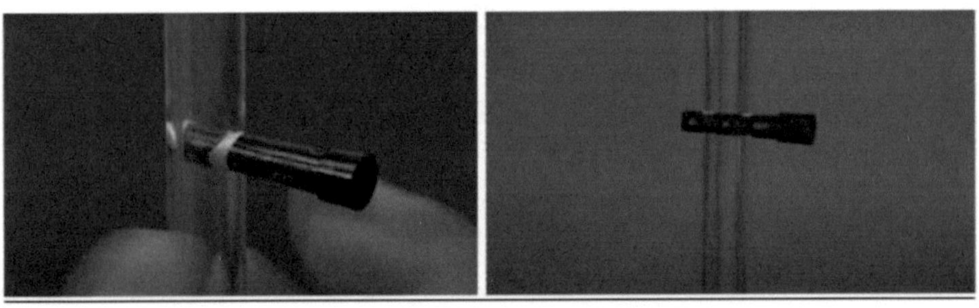

Figure 8.
ID number and bar code of the capsules – in the left. The sensitive area is marked on the capsule – in the right.

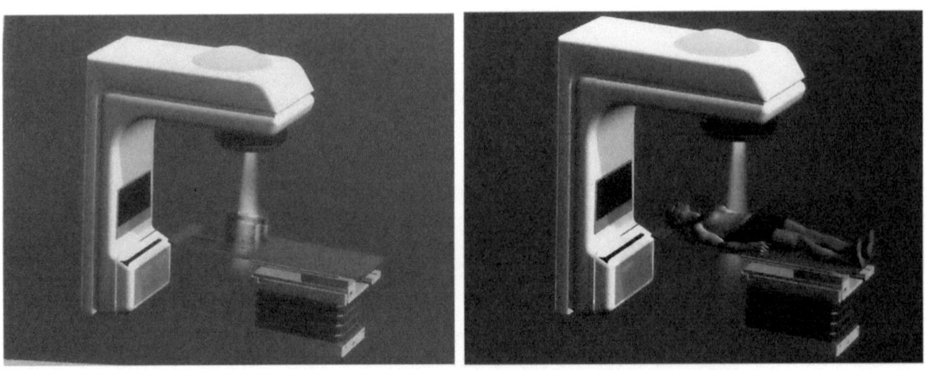

(a) (b)

Figure 9.
The dosimetry audit should be performed in the same conditions in which patient is irradiated during treatment procedure.

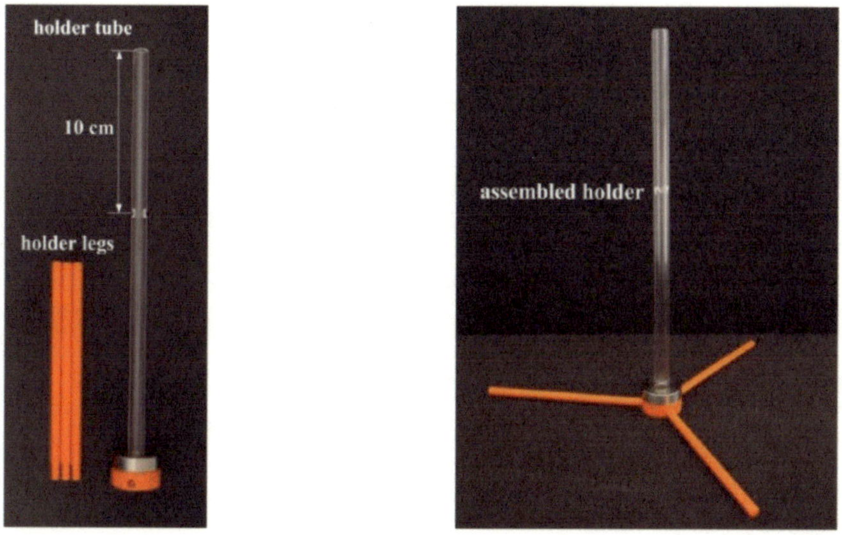

Figure 10.
Assembling the IAEA standard holder for the RPLDs irradiations [25, 26].

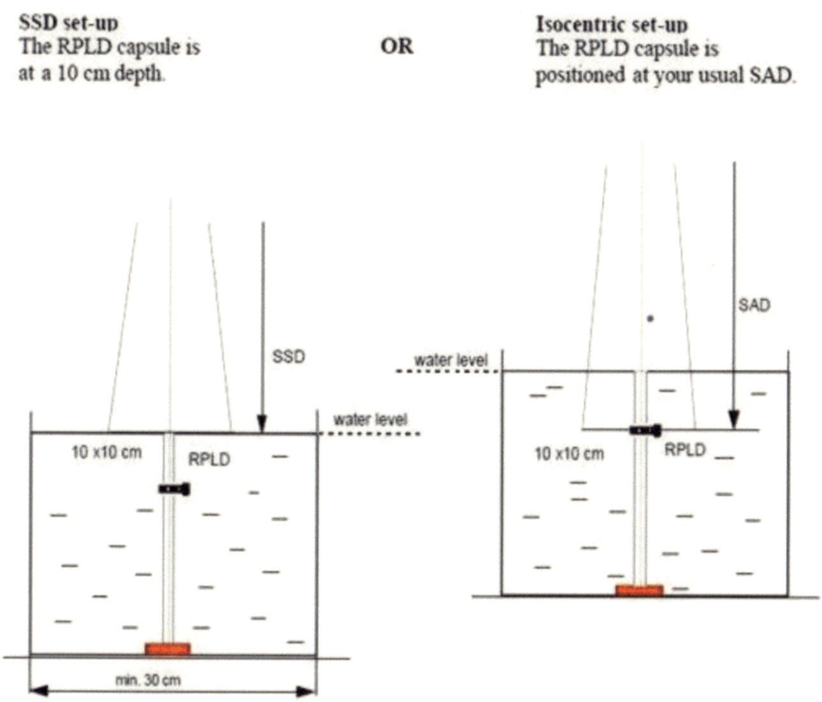

Figure 11.
Two alternative geometry set-ups for the RPLD irradiation [25, 26].

5. Adjust the water level by filling the water tank exactly to the level of the top of the holder. Make sure that the tube of the holder is also filled with water (**Figure 11**).

6. Adjust the patient' couch height so that the water surface is at your usual distance using in the daily clinical practice.

II. Irradiation of the RPLDs.

The procedure of irradiation of the dosimeters covers the following actions:

1. Before irradiation recheck whether the alignment, field size, water level and distance are correct (**Figure 11**).

2. Insert the capsule into the hole of the holder, so that the dot on the capsule is positioned in the centre of the tube (**Figure 12**).

3. Irradiate the RPLD capsule with the number of monitor units (MU) calculated above.

4. Remove the capsule from the holder (**Figure 12**) and wipe it dry.

5. Repeat the procedure, steps 2 to 4, for the second capsule.

The total 2 /two/ RPLD capsules per beam should be irradiated for the purpose of dosimetry audit.

The following recommendations should be taken into account:

1. An RPLD capsule in a small bag must not be irradiated, because it is used to record environmental influences during transport and storage.

2. Calculation of the number of monitor units to deliver 2 Gy to a tumor, whose centre is the RPLD capsule is at 10 cm depth.

The absorbed dose to water D_w is calculated from the RPLD response registered by the RPLD reader according to the expression:

$$D = M.N.SCF.PCF.f_{lin}.f_{fad}.f_{en}.f_{hol}, \quad (1)$$

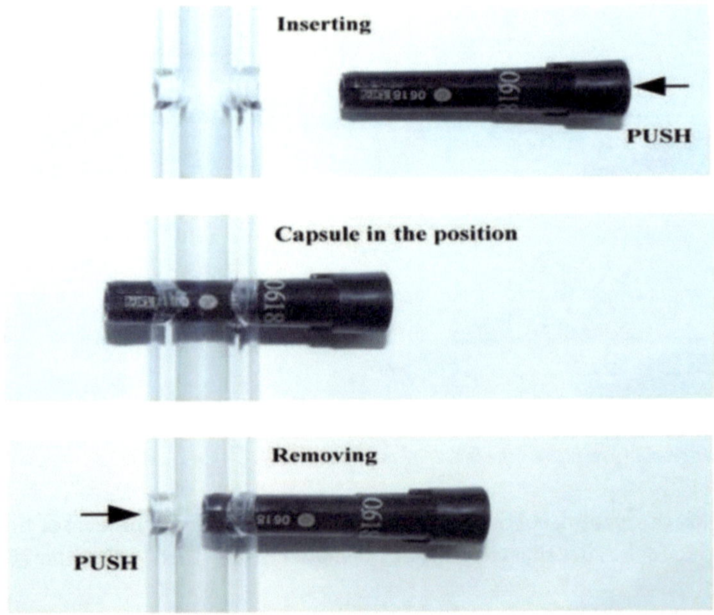

Figure 12.
Different positions of the capsule with RPLD – inserting, capsule in the position and removing [25, 26].

where:

M [counts] – is the RPLD response, the mean of the readings from one dosimeter corrected for the ray readout position.

N [Gy/counts] – is the calibration coefficient of the RPLD system and is defined as the inverse of RPL response per unit dose to water; N is determined for 2 Gy delivery from Co-60 beam.

SCF – is individual sensitivity correction factor.

PCF – is the radiation position correction factor.

$\mathbf{f_{lin}}$ – is the non-linearity dose response correction factor.

$\mathbf{f_{en}}$ - is the energy correction factor.

$\mathbf{f_{fad}}$ – is the fading correction factor.

$\mathbf{f_{hol}}$ – is the standard IAEA RPLD holder correction factor.

The determination of all these factors, their values, meitanence, quality assurance and combined uncertainty of the RPLD system are comprehensively given in [27].

9. Results of dosimetry audit with RPLDs

Bulgarian radiotherapy centres participated in the IAEA/WHO Postal Dose Audit Service with (RPLD) in last three years. The new Varian and Elekta therapy treatment machines have been installed in 2011–2017. The energy of the photon beams is in the range of 6 MV-15 MV. The total number of 34 beams were cheked. The results are given on **Figure 13**. The 33 beams (97%) in reference conditions are in the tolerance of +/– 5%. Follow up have been organized for the beam exceed the tolerance and successfully is clarified the reason. The results of the dosimetry audits despite the fact, that the radiotherapy equipment in Bulgaria was in long-term technology stagnation, show the ability of Bulgarian medical physicists to provide quality dosimetric control at the current world criteria.

The results show, that all measured values of the applied dose are within ±5%. There is a tendency to improve the accuracy, which we attribute to the in-depth

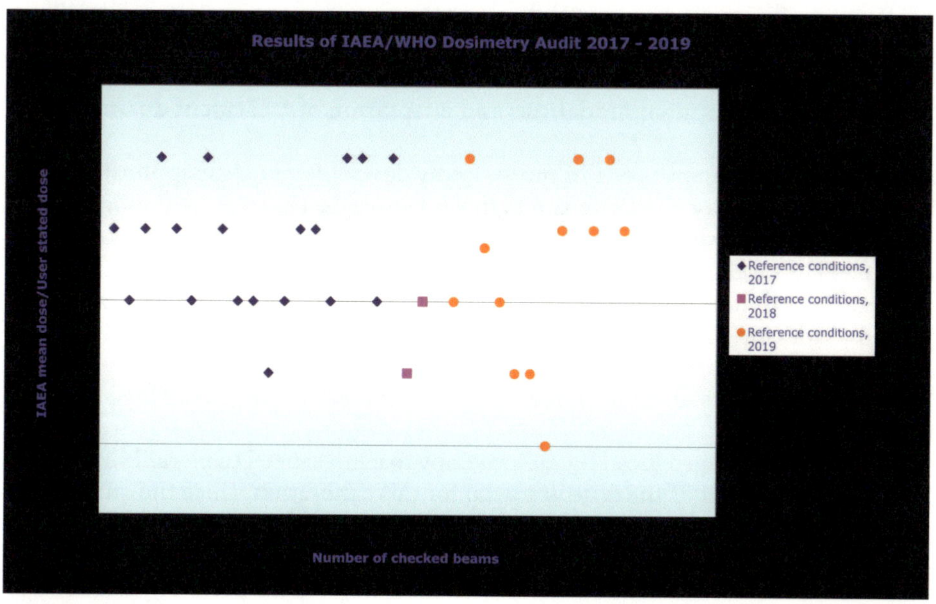

Figure 13.
The results of IAEA/WHO RPLD audit 2017–2019. Ratios of IAEA mean dose/stated dose. Each point in the graph represent averaged dose of 2(two) capsules.

knowledge, experience and skills of the staff of medical physicists due to their regularly participation in the dosimetry audits.

Independent dosimetry audits play an important role in patient treatment quality, radiation protection and safety. Audits have the potential to identify issues and resolve them, reducing the probability of harmful errors to occur. They also support the safe implementation of new techniques and technologies, and promote knowledge sharing at a national and/or international level by benchmarking centres with similar equipment [28]. Indeed, the IAEA stresses the importance of every radiotherapy centre equipped with new machines and those that are going to introduce new treatment techniques in clinical practice, participate in dosimetry audits before starting treating patients, and regularly after that [29]. Moreover, a recent European Directive (2013/59 Euratom) recommends that new radiological procedures should be audited. Independent dose audits are also mandatory in many multi-institutional clinical trials in radiotherapy to ensure that participants deliver accurate doses and so the reported results are not biased [30–32].

10. Discussion

The need of safe and effective radiotherapy is growing as cancer morbidity is growing worldwide. Modern radiotherapy is used to treat and improve the quality of life of patients undergoing this type of therapy. Currently, radiation therapy is widely recognized as one of the safest areas of modern medicine and errors in radiation therapy are very rare [33].

Patient safety is of paramount importance to medical staff in radiotherapy centers and safety considerations are an element in all aspects of the day-to-day clinical activities. Technological advances and clinical research over the past few decades have given radiation oncologists the capability to personalize treatments for accurate delivery of radiation dose based on clinical parameters and anatomical information. Two major strategies, acting synergistically, will enable further widening of the therapeutic window of radiation oncology in the era of precision medicine: technology-driven improvement of treatment conformity, including advanced image guidance and particle therapy, and novel biological concepts for personalized treatment, including biomarker-guided prescription, combined treatment modalities and adaptation of treatment during its course [34].

Modern radiotherapy is one of most rapidly developing nuclear applications in medicine and today it is a safe and highly effective cancer treatment modality. Precise radiation dosimetry measurements are used to keep radiotherapy safe and effective. The need of dosimetric and geometric accuracy in radiotherapy is well defined [28, 35]. Recommendations of the International Commission of Radiation Units and Measurements (ICRU) given as early as in 1976, state that the dose delivery to the primary target should be within ±5% of the prescribed value (but in some special circumstances it should comply within ±2% to the prescribed dose to the target [36].

Radiation beams produced by radiotherapy machines need to be calibrated. Precise measurement of the dose is crucial for this calibration, since the quality and effectiveness of the medical radiation therapy rely on their accuracy. By the end of 2018, 2364 radiotherapy centres in 136 countries world-wide have been audited by the IAEA/WHO; 4427 machines and 5790 beams were encompassed by the audit programme. The total results of 13,756 individual TLD/RPLD irradiated sets over a period of 50 years were readout, evaluated and analyzed. 86% of them are within the 5% acceptance limit [37].

11. Conclusion

In our days, modern radiation therapy requires technologically advanced equipment and a professional strategy for the treatment of cancer patients in order to achieve the best clinical result, especially when the vision of the European Society for Radiation Therapy and Oncology for 2020 is: "Every cancer patient in Europe will have access to state-of-the-art radiation therapy as part of a multidisciplinary approach in which treatment is individualized for a particular patient's cancer, taking into account the patient's personal circumstances" [38].

Professionalism and morality oblige us to provide safe and effective radiation therapy, i.e. to know, that we are doing everything well, but also to be able to do it even better. Times have changed, mostly for the better. Few could argue with the fact that the tools we work with today are extremely superior and extremely complex than a few years ago. Advances in technology provide more sophisticated, promising and accurate techniques for targeting malignancies, while minimizing normal tissue damage is crucial for patients treated with radiation therapy [39].

Dosimetry audit has been identified in the activities of ESTRO as one of the most important topics, accompanying the improvement of the quality of radiotherapy practice in Europe through standardization [28]. International organizations as the IAEA and EU in their recent recommendations place external dosimetry audit as a mandatory element in the quality assurance program in radiotherapy [18, 35].

Over the years, the audits have contributed to good dosimetry practice and accuracy of dose measurements in modern radiotherapy. Dosimetry audit ensures, that the correct therapeutic dose is delivered to the patients undergoing radiotherapy and play a key role in activities to create a good *radiation protection* and *safety culture*. One important component of *safety culture*, particularly in the nuclear applications is radiation safety for employees and local communities, while in radiotherapy means safety of the patients and hospital staff. The newest technologies undoubtedly lead to constant trends in the enhancing of the basic principles of *radiation protection* - justification and optimization and to create a good safety culture allowing us to treat more cancer patients in efficient, effective and safely manner.

Acknowledgements

With acknowledgments to the IAEA for organizing my scientific visit at IAEA Dosimetry Laboratory in October 2019 in connection with Technical Cooperation Project: BUL6014 Establishing a National Dosimetry Audit System and Dosimetry Quality Audit Programme in Radiation Therapy with objective to enhance safer radiation therapy treatment in Bulgaria.

Conflict of interest

The author declare no conflict of interest.

Notes

The author highly appreciate the long-term efforts and activities of IAEA to improve continuously quality of radiotherapy, radiation protection and safety of patients, providing standards, training and guidance, direct technical assistance and building capacity and awareness.

Author details

Katia Manolova Sergieva
Queen Giovanna University Hospital, Sofia Medical University, Sofia, Bulgaria

*Address all correspondence to: sergievakm@abv.bg

References

[1] Available on: https://bg.wikipedia.org/wiki/%D0%9A%D0%BB%D0%B8%D0%BD%D0%B8%D1%87%D0%B5%D0%BD_%D0%BE%D0%B4%D0%B8%D1%82

[2] Available on: https://www.who.int/news-room/fact-sheets/detail/cancer

[3] Abdel-Wahab M, Bourque JM, Pynda Y, et al: Status of radiotherapy resources in Africa: An International Atomic Energy Agency analysis. Lancet Oncol, 2013, 14:e168-e175.

[4] Barton MB, Gebski V, Manderson C, et al: Radiation therapy: Are we getting value for money? Clin Oncol (R Coll Radiol), 1995, 7:287-292.

[5] Atun R, Jaffray DA, Barton MB, et al: Expanding global access to radiotherapy. Lancet Oncol, 2015, 16:1153-1186.

[6] Aruah SC, Asogwa OC, Ubah FI, Maurice NN, Oyesegun R, Ige TA, Coleman CN, Dosanjh M, Pistenmaa D. Overcoming Challenges in Providing Radiation Therapy to Patients With Cancer in Nigeria and Experience in the National Hospital Abuja, Nigeria. JCO Glob Oncol. 2020 Aug;6:1232-1236. doi: 10.1200/JGO.19.00177. PMID: 32755480; PMCID: PMC7456314.

[7] Kum Bae Kim, Sang Hyoun Choi. Postal Dosimetry Audits for the Domestic Medical Linear Accelerator. Progress in Medical Physics 31(2), June 2020. https://doi.org/10.14316/pmp.2020.31.2.20

[8] International Atomic Energy Agency. Accuracy requirements and uncertainties in radiotherapy, human health Series 31. Vienna: IAEA; 2016.

[9] van der Merwe D, Christaki K. IAEA support to radiotherapy dosimetry. Acta Oncol. 2020 May;59(5):493-494. doi: 10.1080/0284186X.2020.1726457. Epub 2020 Feb 14. PMID: 32056484.

[10] Izewska, J., Quality improvement in radiotherapy: history, significance and impact of dosimetry audits, Radiother. Oncol. 123 (2017) 599.

[11] IZEWSKA, J., SVENSSON, H., IBBOTT, G., "Worldwide quality assurance networks for radiotherapy dosimetry", Standards and Codes of Practice in Medical Radiation Dosimetry (Proc. Int. Symp. Vienna, 2002), Vol. 2, IAEA, Vienna (2003) 139-156.

[12] IZEWSKA, J., ANDREO, P., VATNITSKY, S., SHORTT, K.R., The IAEA/WHO TLD postal dose quality audits for radiotherapy: A perspective of dosimetry practices at hospitals in developing countries, Radiother. Oncol. 69 (2003) 91-97.

[13] AGUIRRE, J.F., TAILOR, R., IBBOTT, G., STOVALL, M., HANSON, W., "Thermoluminescence dosimetry as a tool for the remote verification of output for radiotherapy beams: 25 years of experience", Standards and Codes of Practice in Medical Radiation Dosimetry (Proc. Int. Symp. Vienna, 2002), Vol. 2, IAEA, Vienna (2003) 191-199.

[14] Bolt MA, Clark CH, Chen T, Nisbet A. A multi-centre analysis of radiotherapy beam output measurement. Phys Imag Radiat Oncol 2017;4:39-43.

[15] Thwaites D. Accuracy required and achievable in radiotherapy dosimetry: have modern technology and techniques changed our views? J Phys Conf Ser 2013;444:012006.

[16] Followill DS, Evans DR, Cherry C, Molineu A, Fisher G, Hanson WF, et al. Design, development, and implementation of the Radiological

Physics Center's pelvis and thorax anthropomorphic quality assurance phantoms. Med Phys 2007;34:2070.

[17] Izewska J, Azangwe G, Bera P. 40 years of the IAEA/WHO TLD postal dose audits for radiotherapy. SSDL Newsletter No. 58, June 2010, 17-23.

[18] European Parliament. Council Directive 2013/59/Euratom of 5 December 2013 laying down basic safety standards for protection against the dangers arising from exposure to ionising radiation, and repealing Directives 89/618/Euratom, 90/641/ Euratom, 96/29/Euratom, 97/43/ Euratom a. Off J Eur Commun L13 2014:1-73.

[19] Melidis C, Bosch WR, Izewska J, Fidarova E, Zubizarreta E, Ulin K, et al. Global harmonization of quality assurance naming conventions in radiation therapy clinical trials. Int J Radiat Oncol Biol Phys 2014;90:1242-1249. https://doi.org/ 10.1016/j.ijrobp. 2014.08.348.

[20] Oscar Casares-Magaz, Loredana G. Marcu, Yolanda Prezado, Efi Koutsouveli, Marco Brambilla. EFOMP survey results on national radiotherapy dosimetry audits. Physica Medica (IF2.685), Pub Date: 2021-03-31, DOI: 10.1016/j.ejmp.2021.03.020

[21] Takayoshi Yamamoto, RPL Dosimetry: Principles and Applications, AIP Conf. Proc. 1345, 217 (2011); doi: 10.1063/1.3576169. Available on: http:// dx.doi.org/10.1063/1.3576169

[22] Schulman J. H. et al., Dosimetry of X-rays and 7-rays by radiophotoluminescence, J. Appl.Phye., 22, 1479(1951).

[23] Tsuda M., A Few Remarks on Photoluminescence Dosimetry with High Energy X-Rays. Igaku Butsuri. 2000, 20 (3) pp. 131-139.

[24] J. Sempau, P.Kazantsev, J.Izewska, L.Brualla. Monte Carlo verification of the holder correction factors for the radiophotoluminescent glass dosimeter used by the IAEA in international dosimetry audits. Physica Medica, 2021, 86, 1-5.

[25] RPLD Instruction Sheet (English). pdf - Dosimetry Audit Networks. Available on: https://dosimetry-audit-networks.iaea.org

[26] Katia Sergieva. Dosimetry audit in radiotherapy – key role in safety culture. Merit Research Journal of Medicine and Medical Sciences, Vol. 8(8) pp. 448-455, August, 2020.

[27] Joanna Izewska et al. IAEA, DOLP.066. Maintenance of the radiopotoluminescnt (RPL) reference dosimetry system for radiotherapy, 2019.

[28] Clark CH, Jornet N, Muren LP. The role of dosimetry audit in achieving high quality radiotherapy. Phys Imaging Radiat Oncol 2018;5:85-87. doi:10.1016/j. phro.2018.03.009.

[29] International Atomic Energy Agency. Accuracy Requirements and Uncertainties in Radiotherapy. Vienna: IAEA Human Health Series; 2016. doi:10.1038/sj.bjc.6604224.

[30] Ibbott GS, Haworth A, Followill DS. Quality assurance for clinical trials. Front Oncol 2013;3:311. doi:10.3389/ fonc.2013.00311.

[31] Weber DC, Poortmans PMP, Hurkmans CW, Aird E, Gulyban A, Fairchild A. Quality assurance for prospective EORTC radiation oncology trials: the challenges of advanced technology in a multicenter international setting. Radiother Oncol 2011;100:150-156. doi:10.1016/j. radonc.2011.05.073.

[32] Melidis C, Bosch W, Izewska J, Fidarova E, Zubizarreta E, Ishikura S, et al. Radiation therapy quality assurance in clinical trials-Global Harmonisation Group. Radiother Oncol 2014;111. doi:10.1016/j.radonc.2014.03.023.

[33] General guidelines on risk management in external beam radiotherapy, EU, RADIATION PROTECTION N° 181, 2015.

[34] Michael Baumann, Mechthild Krause, Jens Overgaard, et al. Radiation oncology in the era of precision medicine. Nature Reviews Cancer 16, 2016, 234 - 249.

[35] IAEA SAFETY STANDARDS SERIES No. SSG-46. Radiation protection and safety in medical uses of ionizing radiation, International Atomic Energy Agency, Vienna, 2018.

[36] International Commission on Radiation Units and Measurements. Determination of absorbed dose in a patient irradiated by beams of X or gamma rays in radiotherapy procedures. ICRU report 24. Bethesda, MD: IRCU; 1976.

[37] Joanna Izewska et al. 50 Years of the IAEA/WHO postal dose audit programme for radiotherapy: what can we learn from 13756 results? Acta Oncologica 2020, 59(2):1-8. doi.org/10.1080/0284186X.2020.1723162]

[38] Available on: http://www.estro.org/about/mission-values/vision

[39] Katia Sergieva. Trends in radiation protection of patients in modern radiotherapy. IAEA Conference: International Conference on Radiation Protection in Medicine: Achieving Change in Practice At: December 2017, Vienna, Austria. Available on: https://www.researchgate.net/publication/322064907_Trends_in_radiation_protection_of_patients_in_modern_radiotherapy

Chapter 7

Volumetric and Dosimetric Inconstancy of Parotid Glands and Tumor in Head and Neck Cancer during IMRT

Seema Gupta, Shraddha Srivastava, Navin Singh and Arunima Ghosh

Abstract

The treatment of head and neck cancer using external beam radiotherapy is commonly done with three field techniques, which involves bilateral parallel opposed beams and one anterior lower neck field. Conventional treatment is based on 2D fluoroscopic images where there is no facility to shield the organs at risk like parotid. The most common side effect of such conventional radiotherapy treatment is xerostomia. The incidence of radiotherapy-related xerostomia varies depending on the specific radiotherapy technique used and the dose delivered to the parotid glands. Dosimetric variation in the tumor and normal tissue including parotid glands due to volume shrinkage during intensity modulated radiotherapy is the leading challenges in radiotherapy delivery in head and neck malignancy in terms of acute and late radiation related toxicities. Therefore if the planning target volume and normal tissue anatomy are changing with time during intensity modulated radiotherapy, it would be beneficial and acceptable to adapt our treatment delivery to minimize normal tissue toxicities where it really matters.

Keywords: volumetric, dosimetric, parotid glands, head and neck cancer, IMRT

1. Introduction

One of the biggest challenges in radiotherapy delivery in head and neck cancer is radiation related acute and late toxicities. Symptoms of acute toxicities can be present for up to 3 months post-radiotherapy, and late toxicities, tend to persist several months or years after the completion of radiotherapy.

Xerostomia is considered to be a major concern in radiation related acute and late toxicity after head and neck radiotherapy.

2. Radiobiology of parotid glands

Salivary gland cells are slow dividing cells even though they are highly radiosensitive, factors attributing to this could be smaller number of cells in the functional subunit of acinar cells, slow recovery of acinar cells, depletion of stem cell

IntechOpen

population, pattern and rate of terminal differentiation of stem cells, proliferation rate of the stem cells, turn over or life time of acinar cells. If turn over or life time of cell is short there will be early appearance of symptoms of radiation injury and vice versa if the cell turn over or life time of cell is long.

In slowly dividing tissue radiation injury becomes more prominent when dose per fraction is increased, because at higher dose there are fewer division cycles that cells can successfully negotiate before their death. Therefore injury develops more quickly with increase in dose per fraction in late dividing tissue.

Various inter current insults e.g. chemotherapy, surgery, dental or mechanical trauma, hyperthermia, infection are also capable of precipitating the expression of radiation injury in slowly responding tissues.

3. Radiation techniques in head and neck cancers

The treatment of head and neck cancer (HNC) using external beam radiotherapy is commonly done with three field techniques, which involves bilateral parallel opposed beams and one anterior lower neck field. Conventional treatment is based on 2D fluoroscopic images where there is no facility to shield the organs at risk like parotid [1]. The most common side effect of such conventional radiotherapy treatment is xerostomia. This damage to salivary glands causes a reduction in saliva, dryness of mouth, difficulty in chewing, and speech alterations [2, 3]. Dental caries, which results in impaired nutrition, weight loss and significant degradation of quality of life, so their management and prevention is important for radiotherapy. The incidence of radiotherapy-related xerostomia varies depending on the specific radiotherapy technique used and the dose delivered to the parotid glands.

With the advancement in imaging and treatment planning techniques, CT-based conformal radiotherapy has come into existence which delivers radiation to the target with precision and gives minimal dose to the parotids. These techniques involve three-dimensional conformal radiotherapy (3D-CRT), intensity-modulated radiation therapy (IMRT), and volumetric modulated arc therapy (VMAT). The evolution of imaging methods from 2D portals to 3D-CBCT (Cone beam CT) has established the role of image-guided radiotherapy in improving the inter and intra-fractional variations during Radiotherapy of HNC [4]. These high precision techniques have led to an improvement in dose distribution and significant sparing of OARs (in this case parotid) and reduction in radiation-induced xerostomia [1]. The various radiotherapy treatment planning techniques in HNC have been discussed here.

4. Three-dimensional conformal radiotherapy (3D-CRT)

In the 3D-CRT technique for the treatment of HNC, usually, three fields are used. This consists of bilateral portals to treat the primary tumor and cervical lymph nodes and an anterior field to treat lower jugular chain and supraclavicular group of lymph nodes. A total dose of 70 Gy in 35 fractions is delivered in two to three phases in the definitive setting and 60–66 GY in 2 Gy per fraction in the adjuvant setting with or without concurrent chemotherapy depending on indications [5, 6]. Due to large hotspots arising in this technique, Field in field technique or field segmentation is generally used to reduce the hot spots. Monoisocentric technique is generally used where the bilateral and anterior fields have a common isocenter. This removes the problem of beam divergence and field abutment to avoid under dosing of tumor volume and overdosing of critical structures. However, despite the matching of the lower border of bilateral fields and the upper border of the anterior neck field, there is a chance of error in the junction dose due to various dosimetric and physical factors causing inhomogeneity in the dose distribution in that area. The dosimetric factors include field size, beam quality, penumbra etc., while the physical factors include the jaw alignment, isocenter accuracy etc. [7]. Despite, all such efforts, a significant amount of dose is received by OARs (organs at risk) like parotid causing treatment toxicity like xerostomia. This limits the ability of 3D-CRT to spare the OARs when there is a concave-shaped target in the head and neck. Therefore, the 3D-CRT technique is not helpful in parotid sparing and cannot be a replacement for higher precision techniques like IMRT.

5. Intensity-modulated radiotherapy (IMRT)

The 3D-CRT technique is based on the delivery of uniform fluence across the beam and involves less complex beam arrangements. Here, the parameters for planning such as beam directions, beam weights, wedges, etc. are based on the trial and error method making it a time-consuming process. To overcome these challenges, a more sophisticated method of conformal planning known as Intensity-modulated radiotherapy (IMRT) is used in HNC. Unlike the 3D-CRT method, here beams of non-uniform intensity are used. IMRT is based on the principle of inverse planning optimization and uses computed-controlled multi-leaf collimators to modulate the intensity of beams across the tumor. Intensity modulation allows the conformal dose coverage to the target and sharp dose fall-off beyond the target thus sparing the critical structures surrounding the target [8].

Due to the complex anatomy of the head and neck, and proximity of various critical structures with the target, IMRT is the better choice of treatment [9]. Multiple beams of non-uniform intensity deliver dose with high conformity to the irregularly shaped target and steep dose gradient at the boundary of target and organs at risk (OARs) minimize the dose to adjacent OARs like spinal cord, parotids.

Head and neck tumor configurations are usually concave in nature. With multiple organs such as the parotid glands, brainstem, spinal cord etc. surrounding such concave-shaped lesions, there is a need for concave-shaped dose distribution to avoid risking dose to these OARs [10]. Head and neck IMRT clearly offers such advantages of better normal tissue sparing, improved dose coverage to the target, giving multiple isodose levels in tumor volume, and dose -escalation to the tumor [11].

IMRT has given better results over 3D-CRT in head and neck cancer with a significant reduction in xerostomia, prevention of acute and late toxicities, and improved quality of life. Parotid-sparing IMRT has superior results over conventional 3D-CRT [12–14]. However, for successful results from IMRT, there is a requirement of precision in the patient setup, immobilization, and correct tumor volume delineation to avoid any marginal miss, proper plan evaluation, strict imaging protocols, and rigorous quality assurance tests. Owing to the tight margins of dose around the target, any negligence during the IMRT treatment can pose a serious risk to the patient and can impact the treatment outcome. Another concern that arises during IMRT treatment is the volumetric and spatial changes in tumor volume and OARs due to shrinking of tumor, weight loss, radiation-induced toxicities as well as variation due to physiological movements like breathing [15–26] (**Table 1**). One such change observed during treatment of HNC is the movement

Reference	N	Imaging	Anatomic changes	Dosimetric changes
Ho et al. [15]	10	Weekly CBCT	Parotid: V ↓ 25%	Parotid, SC, BS: no change Larynx, OC: no change
Robar et al. [16]	15	Weekly CT	Parotid: V ↓ 4.9%/ week; 0.85 mm/week medial shift	Parotid: Dmean↑ 2.6% (L) SC: ↑ 0.2% BS: ↑ 1.0%
Hunter et al. [17]	18	Daily CBCT	Parotid: V ↓ 13%	Parotid: Dmean↑ 0.9 Gy
Jin et al. [18]	10	Weekly CBCT	Parotid: 4.5-4.7%/ week	Parotid: V26 ↑ 7.5% (R); V26 ↑ 8.8% (L)
Wu et al. [19]	11	Weekly CT	Parotid: V ↓ 15% CTV: V ↓ 10%	Parotid:Dmean↑10% CTV, BS, SC: No change
Bhide et al. [20]	20	Weekly CT		Parotid: Dmean↑ 7% (ipsi) SC: Dmax↑ 2% BS: Dmax↑ 4% PTV1: Dmin↓ 3% PTV2: Dmin↓ 5%
Castadot et al. [21]	10	4 rpt CTs		Parotid: Dmean↑ 4% SC: D2% ↑ 4.5% CTV: No change
Nishi et al. [22]	20	Rpt CT	GTV: V ↓ 63% (primary); V ↓ 52% (nodal) Parotid: V ↓ 18%; 4.2mm medial shift	GTV: D98 ↑ 1% (primary); D98 ↓ 0.3% (nodal) Parotid: Dmean↑20%; SC: D2 ↑ 5%
Castelli et al. [23]	15	Weekly CT		Parotid: Dmean↑ 3.7 Gy (59% parotids)
Barker et al. [24]	14	3 CT per week	Parotid: V ↓ 8% (0.6%/day); 3.1 mm medial shift GTV: V ↓ 70% (1.8%/ day)	
Lee et al. [25]	10	Daily MVCT	Parotid: V ↓ 21% (0.7%/day); 2.6 mm medial shift	
Vásquez Osorio et al. [26]	10	Repeat CT	Parotid: V ↓ 17% (ipsi); V ↓ 5% (contra) SMG: V ↓ 20% (ipsi); V ↓ 11% (contra)	

Abbreviations: SC = spinal cord; BS = brainstem; SMG = submandibular gland; L = left; R = right; V = volume; ipsi = ipsilateral; contra = contralateral.

Table 1.
Summary of anatomic and dosimetric changes throughout treatment for head and neck radiotherapy.

of parotid closer to high dose regions during the progress of treatment owing to the shrinkage in tumor volume, inducing high-grade xerostomia (even worse than predicted) [27]. To limit the dose variation due to these factors, there is a need to adapt to the varying treatment volume and OAR volumes changing during the course of treatment (**Figures 1–4**). This could be possible through a technique known as adaptive radiotherapy.

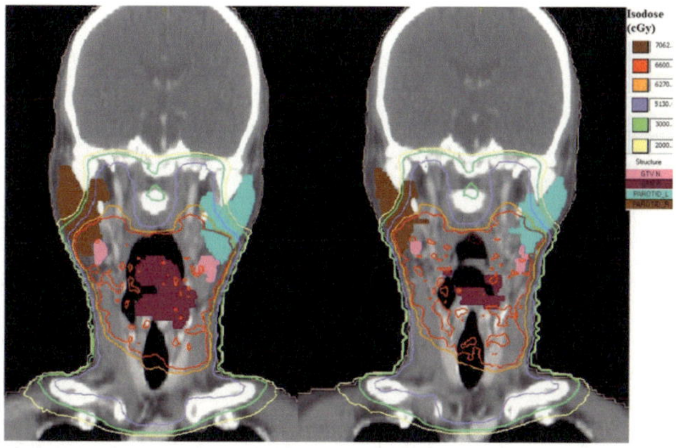

Figure 1.
Comparison between pre-treatment (CT1) [left] and per-treatment (CT4) [right] images of a patient. Coronal CT slices of a 57 years old male patient with carcinoma hypopharynx (T4aN2c). The decrease in volume of GTV primary (maroon) [from 30.426 cc in CT 1 to 5.964 cc in CT 4] and GTV nodal (pink) [from 10.005 cc in CT 1 to 4.638 cc in CT 4] can be appreciated along with decrease in volume of both right (brown) and left (light blue) parotid glands.

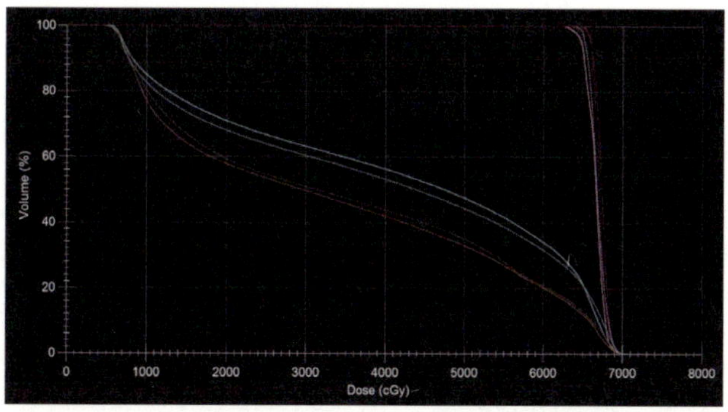

Figure 2.
Comparative DVH of a patient [(Ca hypopharynx T4N2c)] comparing CT1 (-------) and CT4 (——). The mean dose to the right parotid (brown) has decreased in CT4 compared to CT1 whereas the mean dose to left parotid (light blue) has increased in CT4 compared to CT1.

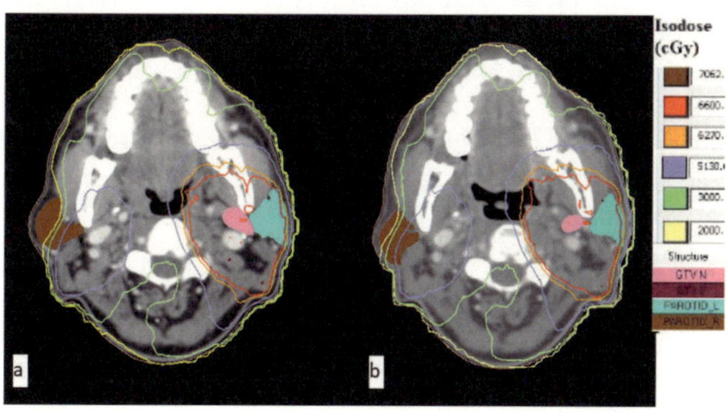

Figure 3.
Comparison between pre-treatment (a) and per-treatment (b) images of a Patient undergoing IMRT-SIB. Coronal CT slices of a 55 years old male carcinoma pyriform fossa (T1N3b) patient. We can appreciate the decrease in GTV nodal (pink) volume by end of treatment along with decrease in volume of both right (brown) and left (light blue) parotid glands (b). The low dose isodose curves of 20 Gy (light yellow) and 30 Gy (light green) can be seen covering more areas of right parotid gland in (b) compared to (a).

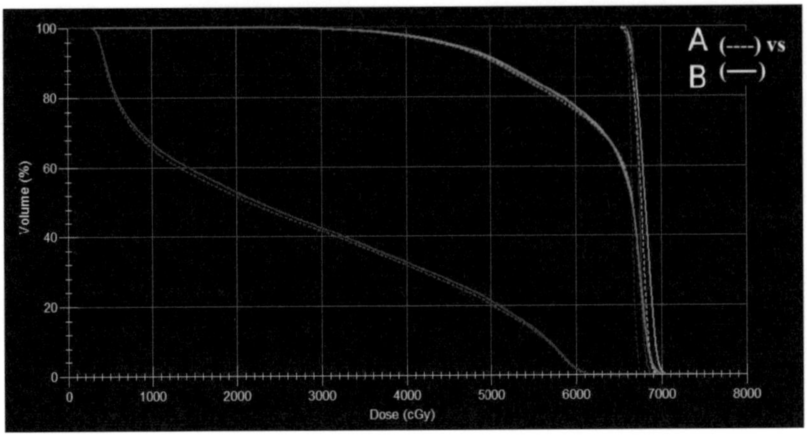

Figure 4.
DVH comparison between start (A) [--------] and end of treatment (B) [———].

6. Adaptive radiotherapy

Adaptive radiotherapy is a technique in which any volumetric or spatial variations in tumor volume or OARs, the morphological changes are taken into account through re-planning of patients at certain defined intervals during the course of treatment. The re-planning helps in adapting to the anatomical changes in tumor and OARs such as parotids and optimizing the plan to provide adequate tumor coverage and minimize the dose to OARs [28]. These variations are corrected on a daily basis through modifications in the treatment plan with the help of image guidance. Routine in-room volumetric images are acquired and sent to the treatment planning system for re-planning. The contours of the daily in-room CT are superimposed with the reference planning CT to account for any variation in the anatomy or set up, through deformable image registration software. A new treatment plan conforming to the current changes in anatomy, if any, is generated through automated deformable registration software and the adapted plan is transferred to the machine for treatment. The new plan is implemented either in online mode after online correction or in offline mode, where the corrections are implemented after some time [29]. Adaptive radiotherapy has offered dosimetric benefits in HNC and its clinical benefits have also been proven by a few studies [30].

Therefore medical fraternity now has a better understanding of radiation related toxicities in head and neck cancers, so it is truly gratifying to deliver radiotherapy by such innovative techniques where it really matters.

Author details

Seema Gupta*, Shraddha Srivastava, Navin Singh and Arunima Ghosh
Department of Radiotherapy, King George's Medical University,
Lucknow, Uttar Pradesh, India

*Address all correspondence to: seemaguptart@gmail.com

References

[1] Gupta T, Sinha S, Ghosh-Laskar S, Budrukkar A, Mummudi N, Swain M, et al. Intensity-modulated radiation therapy versus three-dimensional conformal radiotherapy in head and neck squamous cell carcinoma: Long-term and mature outcomes of a prospective randomized trial. Radiation Oncology. 2020;**15**(1):218

[2] Eisbruch A, Ship JA, Martel MK, Ten Haken RK, Marsh LH, Wolf GT, et al. Parotid gland sparing in patients undergoing bilateral head and neck irradiation: Techniques and early results. International Journal of Radiation Oncology, Biology, Physics. 1996;**36**(2):469-480

[3] Maes A, Weltens C, Flamen P, Lambin P, Bogaerts R, Liu X, et al. Preservation of parotid function with uncomplicated conformal radiotherapy. Radiotherapy and Oncology. 2002;**63**(2):203-211

[4] Sterzing F, Engenhart-Cabillic R, Flentje M, Debus J. Image-guided radiotherapy. A new dimension in radiation oncology. Deutsches Arzteblatt International. 2011;**108**(16):274-280

[5] El-Sayed S, Nelson N. Adjuvant and adjunctive chemotherapy in the management of squamous cell carcinoma of the head and neck region. A meta-analysis of prospective and randomized trials. Journal of Clinical Oncology. 1996;**14**(3):838-847

[6] Olmi P, Crispino S, Fallai C, Torri V, Rossi F, Bolner A, et al. Locoregionally advanced carcinoma of the oropharynx: Conventional radiotherapy vs. accelerated hyperfractionated radiotherapy vs. concomitant radiotherapy and chemotherapy—A multicenter randomized trial. International Journal of Radiation Oncology, Biology, Physics. 2003;**55**(1):78-92

[7] Abdel-Hakim K, Nishimura T, Takai M, Sakahara H. Review of monoisocentric split-field technique for conventional and IMRT treatment in head and neck cancers: Technical limitations and approaches for optimization. Technology in Cancer Research & Treatment. 2005;**4**(1):107-113

[8] Yeh S-A. Radiotherapy for head and neck cancer. Seminars in Plastic Surgery. 2010;**24**(2):127-136

[9] Fu KK, Pajak TF, Trotti A, Jones CU, Spencer SA, Phillips TL, et al. A radiation therapy oncology group (RTOG) phase III randomized study to compare hyperfractionation and two variants of accelerated fractionation to standard fractionation radiotherapy for head and neck squamous cell carcinomas: First report of RTOG 9003. International Journal of Radiation Oncology, Biology, Physics. 2000;**48**:7-16

[10] The International Commission on Radiation Units and Measurements. Journal of the ICRU. 2010;**10**(1):Report 83

[11] Daly-Schveitzer N, Juliéron M, Gan Tao Y, Moussier A, Bourhis J. Intensity-modulated radiation therapy (IMRT): Toward a new standard for radiation therapy of head and neck cancer? European Annals of Oto-rhino-laryngology, Head and Neck diseases. 2011;**128**(5):241-247

[12] Nutting CM, Morden JP, Harrington KJ, Urbano TG, Bhide SA, Clark C, et al. Parotid-sparing intensity modulated versus conventional radiotherapy in head and neck cancer (PARSPORT): A phase 3 multicentre randomised controlled trial. The Lancet Oncology. 2011;**12**(2):127-136

[13] Scott-Brown M, Miah A, Harrington K, Nutting C. Evidence-based review: Quality of life following head and neck intensity-modulated radiotherapy. Radiotherapy and Oncology. 2010;**97**(2):249-257

[14] Jensen SB, Pedersen AML, Vissink A, Andersen E, Brown CG, Davies AN, et al. A systematic review of salivary gland hypofunction and xerostomia induced by cancer therapies: Prevalence, severity and impact on quality of life. Supportive Care in Cancer. 2010;**18**(8):1039-1060

[15] Ho KF, Marchant T, Moore C, Webster G, Rowbottom C, Penington H, et al. Monitoring dosimetric impact of weight loss with kilovoltage (KV) cone beam CT (CBCT) during parotid-sparing IMRT and concurrent chemotherapy. International Journal of Radiation Oncology, Biology, Physics. 2012;**82**(3):e375-e382

[16] Robar JL, Day A, Clancey J, Kelly R, Yewondwossen M, Hollenhorst H, et al. Spatial and dosimetric variability of organs at risk in head-and-neck intensity-modulated radiotherapy. International Journal of Radiation Oncology, Biology, Physics. 2007;**68**(4):1121-1130

[17] Hunter KU et al. Parotid glands dose-effect relationships based on their actually delivered doses: Implications for adaptive replanning in radiation therapy of head-and-neck cancer. International Journal of Radiation Oncology, Biology, Physics. 2013;**87**(4):676-682

[18] Jin X et al. CBCT-based volumetric and dosimetric variation evaluation of volumetric modulated arc radiotherapy in the treatment of nasopharyngeal cancer patients. Radiation Oncology. 2013;**8**:279

[19] Wu Q et al. Adaptive replanning strategies accounting for shrinkage in head and neck IMRT. International Journal of Radiation Oncology, Biology, Physics. 2009;**75**(3):924-932

[20] Bhide SA, Davies M, Burke K, McNair HA, Hansen V, Barbachano Y, et al. Weekly volume and dosimetric changes during chemoradiotherapy with intensity-modulated radiation therapy for head and neck cancer: A prospective observational study. International Journal of Radiation Oncology, Biology, Physics. 2010;**76**(5):1360-1368

[21] Castadot P, Geets X, Lee JA, Grégoire V. Adaptive functional image-guided IMRT in pharyngo-laryngeal squamous cell carcinoma: Is the gain in dose distribution worth the effort? Radiotherapy and Oncology. 2011;**101**(3):343-350

[22] Nishi T, Nishimura Y, Shibata T, Tamura M, Nishigaito N, Okumuraet M. Volume and dosimetric changes and initial clinical experience of a two-step adaptive intensity modulated radiation therapy (IMRT) scheme for head and neck cancer. Radiotherapy and Oncology. 2013;**106**(1):85-89

[23] Castelli J, Simon A, Louvel G, Henry O, Chajon E, Nassef M, et al. Impact of head and neck cancer adaptive radiotherapy to spare the parotid glands and decrease the risk of xerostomia. Radiation Oncology. 2015;**10**:6

[24] Barker JL et al. Quantification of volumetric and geometric changes occurring during fractionated radiotherapy for head-and-neck cancer using an integrated CT/linear accelerator system. International Journal of Radiation Oncology, Biology, Physics. 2004;**59**(4):960-970

[25] Lee C, Langen KM, Weiguo L, Haimerl J, Schnarr E, Ruchala KJ, et al. Evaluation of geometric changes of parotid glands during head and neck cancer radiotherapy using daily MVCT

and automatic deformable registration. Radiotherapy and Oncology. 2008;**89**(1):81-88

[26] Vásquez Osorio EM et al. Local anatomic changes in parotid and submandibular glands during radiotherapy for oropharynx cancer and correlation with dose, studied in detail with nonrigid registration. International Journal of Radiation Oncology, Biology, Physics. 2008;**70**(3):875-882

[27] Naveen BS, GNS N. The necessity of replanning during the intensity-modulated radiotherapy (IMRT) for head and neck cancer, to ensure adequate coverage of target volume. International Journal of Medical Research and Review. 2020;**8**(2):189-100

[28] Morgan HE, Sher DJ. Adaptive radiotherapy for head and neck cancer. Cancers Head & Neck. 2020;**5**:1

[29] Schwartz DL, Dong L. Adaptive radiation therapy for head and neck cancer—Can an old goal evolve into a new standard? Journal of Oncology. 2011;**2011**:690595

[30] Chen AM, Daly ME, Cui J, Mathai M, Benedict S, Purdy JA. Clinical outcomes among patients with head and neck cancer treated by intensity-modulated radiotherapy with and without adaptive replanning. Head & Neck. 2014;**36**(11):1541-1546